Practical Aromatherapy

An explanation of aromatherapy, how it can help restore and maintain health and how to use essential oils to good effect on yourself and others.

Practical Aromatherapy

How to Use Essential Oils to Restore Vitality

by

Shirley Price

*Photographs and illustrations by
Leonard Price*

THORSONS PUBLISHERS LIMITED
Wellingborough, Northamptonshire

First published 1983
Fourth Impression 1985

British Library Cataloguing in Publication Data

Price, Shirley
  Practical Aromatherapy.
  1. Essences and essential oils – Therapeutic use
  I. Title
  615'.32   RS164

  ISBN 0-7225-0805-0

Printed and bound in Great Britain

Contents

Introduction

Aromatherapy is a treatment designed to help by the correct use and application of essential oils obtained from plants. The word 'aroma' means a fragrance or sweet smell, a subtle pervasive quality, the fragrance in plants, spices and other substances, and 'therapy' means a treatment designed to cure.

As the fragrance in a plant *is* its essential oil it is easy to see that aromatherapy is a treatment using essential oils. But knowing what aromatherapy is is only the beginning. In order to understand thoroughly the full meaning it is necessary first to discover and learn about the origins and power of essential oils themselves, and then to learn the various treatments by which the oils can be effectively used.

What Are Essential Oils?
Every living thing has a life force, energy or 'soul' which it is impossible to get hold of or to see. It is this life force which, in human beings, is so wonderful and awe inspiring when we stop to consider the amazing facts about our bodies. It is this life force which is there even when our bodies are in poor health, giving us the strength to try to regain normal health.

The life force of a plant is also something that cannot be seen or touched, but it has been said that it is contained in the essential oil of a plant. It is the 'heart' of a plant and is present in only very, very small quantities, sometimes as little as .01 per cent. It is this life force of the plant which we introduce into the body by aromatherapy, and each oil has its own curative effect on certain parts of the body and its systems.

It has been said that essential oils are actually the hormones of the plants. This is easy to believe, because the hormones *we* produce during our whole life time, and without which we cannot live, are present in very, very small quantities also, and would only fill a thimble! Similarly, it would take at least ten large buckets full of orange blossoms to extract a mere thimbleful of neroli essential oil. And, as our glands produce various hormones which affect our bodily systems, so the plant hormones are capable of giving different effects, when used correctly.

Because of this seemingly mystical quality, many people in this century were sceptical about the medical effects of plant oils. But, apart from the known facts of history, when plants and their essences were the only available remedies for disease, a lot of research has been conducted recently by doctors and chemists, and the results have shown that the ancients knew what they were doing!

Background of Aromatherapy
The history of the use of aromatic oils on the body goes back at least 2,000 years before Christ. There are records in the Bible of the use of plants and their oils, both in the treatment of illness and for religious purposes. The Egyptians used them widely, both as cosmetics and for embalming their dead in order to delay decomposition. They were known in China perhaps even before that time, then their use gradually spread to the Greeks and Romans, who of course brought the idea to Britain.

The earliest written record of their use in England was in the thirteenth century, and from that time a great increase was shown both in oils produced and treatments carried out. Glove makers used to perfume their gloves with essential oils to mask the body odour of the wearer, and it was a known fact that, in the Middle Ages, in times of cholera and other diseases, the perfumers very rarely succumbed to illness. This was because nearly all essential oils are good antiseptics. Nicholas Culpeper's book on herbs, recently reprinted, was originally written in 1652, and his work contains detailed medicinal properties of hundreds of plants.

However, in the nineteenth century, chemists began to produce chemical copies of essential oils; much cheaper to make, but effective only as perfumes and not as treatments. There then followed experiments with chemicals to try and imitate the medicinal properties of the oils, and gradually these were so successful that plants and their therapeutic qualities were in danger of becoming extinct.

Nevertheless, the early twentieth century brought a renewed interest in natural products and treatments, perhaps because many of the synthetic drugs had unwanted side effects, and now pure essential oils, which have no such drawback, are used extensively in foods and toiletries as well as in medicines.

A chemist called Gattefosse (who wrote the first modern book on aromatherapy) discovered, while experimenting with cosmetics, a wonderful healer of burns. Carrying out some tests he burnt his hand rather badly. He had essential oil of lavender in his laboratory and plunged his hand into the pure essence. The burn healed in a very short time – a matter of hours – leaving no scar. He also experimented on soldiers' wounds (during World War I) and discovered oils which greatly accelerated the healing process.

His work revealed that it was possible for essential oils to penetrate the skin and, via the extra-cellular liquids, reach the blood and lymph, which in turn carried them in the circulation to the organs. This whole process varies in each individual, taking as little as half an hour in some people and as long as twelve hours in others. Actual skin penetration takes only a matter of minutes.

Dr Jean Valnet, a French physician, also experimented with essential oils, and treated many of his patients by this method. His book on aromatherapy is now available in an English translation. One of his favourite treatments was the use of essential oils in compresses on the affected part, because of the great penetrative powers which the oils possess. He once treated a young adult (who had scars from a scald in his childhood) by this method, and the scars reduced so considerably after several treatments that they were hardly noticeable.

Madame Maury, who died a few years ago (and whose husband was a notable homoeopath) was a biochemist with an interest in beauty therapy. She also carried out research with essential oils, and developed the massage techniques of aromatherapy, leaving the internal and other methods of use to homoeopathic doctors.

She was eventually persuaded to come to England, where she set up an aromatherapy clinic in London. She also taught the subject, and through Madame Maury passing on her knowledge, many beauty therapists now practise aromatherapy, and several eminent people teach it to qualified beauticians and physiotherapists as a further training subject.

1.

Aromatherapy and You

In ancient times, in the East, people visited their 'physician' not when they were ill, but when they were *well*. If they became ill just after the visit and the physician hadn't foreseen the illness, they didn't pay the bill! Physicians then were mainly acupuncturists, and *kept* the bodily systems in health by regular treatment of all the pressure points on the body, thus ensuring good blood and lymph circulation.

This theory still holds good. If we could keep our blood circulating freely, and the lymph moving at its correct speed round the body, illness would be greatly reduced.

But how many of us have a perfect circulatory system? And why not?

Because, somehow, we all manage to produce tension of some sort in our bodies, either physical of emotional. Not only does modern living lessen the amount of exercise we give our muscles, but we sit with our spines bent, we walk incorrectly, and when we stand we let our weight go first on one leg and then the other.

The effect of this is that the muscles are working overtime to keep us in our 'slovenly' positions; tissues and organs are pushed into the wrong place, pressure is applied where it shouldn't be, and the result of all this is that the blood and lymph have greater difficulty in flowing round evenly, and the toxins and waste carried by the venous and lymphatic systems cannot be eliminated quickly enough by natural means, so therefore they escape into the tissues, causing disturbances in the bodily systems and organs.

The emotional tensions we suffer from bring much more serious consequences. Heart and blood pressure symptoms, sometimes due to incorrect diet, are more often brought about by tension due to such things as traffic (this affects us more than is realized if it is a daily double trip through a large city) or the pressure of work, or the day to day worries which some people cannot seem able to deal with in a relaxed manner.

The other effect on the blood circulation is simply the ageing process. In youth, while we are growing, the body cells are constantly dying and being renewed in every single part of the body; every cell of every bone, muscle, nerve and every drop of blood is continually being replaced, therefore all the organs, including the skin, go through this never ending process of renewal.

As we get older the dead skin cells take longer to be thrown off and longer then to be absorbed (or rejected – in the case of skin) and the new cells take longer to form and grow. This slowing down of the regeneration of cell tissue shows itself by a slowing down of all bodily functions, loss of energy, possible constipation, muscles without good tone, loose and often sallow skin.

It is now generally accepted that our state of mind can affect the state of our body, and many illnesses today have a psychosomatic origin. The mind is the most important part of us, yet it is the one thing we cannot touch or even X-ray. It is responsible for our feelings; love, hate, generosity, selfishness, anger, fear, embarrassment, frustration – what a long list of components there are that make up the mind.

Plant hormones, or essential oils, have much the same effect on us, except that they have first to be chosen to suit the emotional upset, and then be applied and hence absorbed into the bloodstream.

If the art of relaxation can be practised, whether by yoga, mind dynamics or by hypnotherapy, then the mind itself can be strengthened in positive application, and a better life can be lived by the owner of that mind, positively affecting both career and health.

Given belief in ourselves – practically anything is possible; it is known that *determination* to succeed is almost inevitably followed by success, in just the same way that determination not to succumb to the common cold will almost inevitably send it away with only the mildest of symptoms. It is no use trying to help someone who does not believe in the method of help used, because their mind has automatically put up a negative barrier.

People already convinced about natural products are more prepared to believe that brown bread is better for health than white bread, than someone who thinks health food eaters are just cranks; bread is just bread and white tastes better anyway!

By making a conscious effort at a quiet time in each day to relax, and train our minds to run only in *positive* channels leading to success and health, we can greatly minimize the negative channels, which only lead to physical and mental disease.

Finally, the other aspect of living which affects our bodily and mental health is our *diet*. Eating a lot of artificially prepared foods containing chemical additives is not conducive to good health or clear skin. The skin reflects the condition of the body, which in turn gives us an idea of the state of mind. No skin preparations, natural or otherwise, will improve the texture or appearance of a blemished skin so long as unsuitable foods are continually being eaten.

Unnatural (i.e., refined and artificially processed) foods are a contributory factor to ill-health, as much as physical and mental stress. With this type of diet we are putting the digestive system under tension, too many rich foods can lead to troubles in the gall bladder or stomach.

Too much sugar (white, refined) and animal fat is often said to contribute to heart disease. The organs of elimination become congested because too many refined starchy foods are eaten, with not enough roughage, and this in itself can cause malfunctions within our systems.

What a sad story!!

However, all these harmful effects can be considerably minimized if we can keep our blood circulation as healthy as possible. Unaided we can see that we eat only the correct foods and not too much of them! (The recent high-fibre diet is an excellent example of giving the roughage needed to keep the bodily systems in good order, and one can eat a lot yet lose weight with this diet, too!)

When the mind is at peace, we experience only positive feelings like love, contentment, selflessness, generosity, etc., and our body responds by being healthy. At other times anger, fear, jealousy, selfishness and depression dominate, and these adversely affect the state of the body. Hormones are released automatically to cope with these feelings and try to return them to a positive state as quickly as possible.

We can make sure that we not only get plenty of exercise, but also re-educate ourselves in the art of sitting, standing and moving correctly. The trouble is that these things need a conscious effort of will, and we have to be really keen and interested to persevere until it simply becomes a habit.

Nonetheless, there is another way to help ourselves, and this is by the use of essential oils.

We tend to wait these days until we are showing symptoms of illness before going to be treated, whereas prevention is, and always will be, better than cure. Aromatherapy is a very good way of *keeping* healthy, and should be used as a preventative treatment in the same way as the Chinese used acupuncture centuries ago.

Methods of getting essential oils into the blood stream (other than by taking them internally) are by baths, inhalations, compresses and various types of massage, varying from simple effleurage through to more advanced forms such as lymph drainage, neuro-muscular technique and shiatsu (where the acupressure points on the meridian lines are used.)

Aromatherapy Body Massage

Regular aromatherapy treatments from a qualified person will bring about, and retain for much longer, a dramatic improvement in well-being and general health, increased vitality and a visible improvement in the texture and colour of the skin.

Every treatment is individual – no two people are exactly the same, and many factors must be taken into consideration when deciding on the form the treatment will take, and the oils that will be used.

Essential oils are extremely concentrated. One drop in 10 to 20 ml of carrier oil will give an identifying aroma, and in fact the true aroma of the plant is obtained by the correct dilution of the essence. Essential oils in their natural state give off too strong an aroma to be pleasant, and this is an important fact to consider. Each one gives off its own peculiar waves, affecting different people in various ways. From the nose a message is sent to the brain, and either pleasure or distaste results as the brain interprets the message.

Our olfactory nerves play a very big part in the success of the treatment so the oils chosen must, when blended in the carrier oil, have an aroma that is pleasing. If the person doesn't like the fragrance it is necessary to find other oils which have the same therapeutic effect but are more appealing aesthetically.

A good aromatherapist will blend oils taking into consideration the volatility, the effects on the bodily or mental conditions, and also the effect of the aroma on the person being treated. This last, as mentioned earlier, is of equal importance to the other two, when essential oils are being used in a specialized aromatherapy massage.

It is important, and interesting, to note that after an

aromatherapy massage the oil should never be washed off, and a bath or shower should not be taken until six to eight hours after treatment, to ensure full absorption of the essential oils (even though they appear to have penetrated fully).

Should there not be an aromatherapist in your area it is possible to help yourself at home by using essential oils in various ways, all of which will be dealt with in detail in the following chapters.

2.

Essential Oils

A lot has been said about essential oils so far, but without mentioning how they are obtained, what the various oils will do, or how the oils themselves vary in quality.

Earlier, the mystical quality of essential oils was mentioned – the life force or personality of the plant. This quality varies during each day or season, and this naturally affects the oil itself. The explanation for this is that during the life of the plant the essential oil cells (distributed throughout the leaves, flowers, stems, bark or root in minute odiferous droplets) change their chemical composition according to the time of day or the season of the year.

It is therefore important to gather herbs and plants for therapeutic use, or distillation into essential oils, at exactly the right time – not so easy in these days of regular working hours!

Many flowers have a heavier and more effective aroma at dusk, and jasmine oil, one of the most expensive oils to buy, produces a higher percentage of essential oil with the richest aroma (and therefore the best theraputic effect) at sunset.

Ylang-ylang blossoms all the year round, but the May and June flowers yield the highest percentage of essential oil.

The amount of oil present in plants varies considerably; in some it is as little as .01 per cent which makes the resultant concentrate very expensive; in some it is as much as 10 per cent, which results in a reasonably priced oil.

A producer of essential oils also has to take into consideration loss of oil by evaporation once the plant is picked and is being transported to the distillery. In the east they still distil lemongrass and one or two other grasses on the spot, usually in a portable copper still which they set up by the stream where the plants are growing. This way they get maxiumum oil yield.

Other factors which influence the quality and yield of essential oil in a plant are the different soil conditions in which they are grown and the variations in climate of different countries; e.g., French jasmine, English lavender and Arabian rose are the most expensive oils of their type.

Essential oils are usually secreted from special glands, ducts or cells in one or several parts of aromatic plants, and from the sap and tissues of certain trees. They are present in the roots, stems, barks, leaves and/or flowers in varying quantities, and in certain botanical families they are more abundant than in others, for example:

Conifarae – which speaks for itself,

Myrtaceae – which family includes eucalyptus, and

Labiatae – to which all mints belong, and which has among its members the useful aromatic plants of lavender, peppermint and rosemary.

The more oil glands or ducts present in the plant, the cheaper the final cost of the oil, and oils from plants with few oil producing glands are necessarily more expensive, for example:

100 kilos of eucalyptus yields about 10 litres of oil.

100 kilos of some varieties of lavender plants can yield almost 3 litres of oil.

100 kilos of some varieties of rose petals can give a yield of up to ½ litre of oil.

So we discover that the cost of producing essential oils is not only in direct proportion to the quality of the plant, as stated earlier, but is also dependent on the quantity of oil-producing glands present in the plant.

An essential oil can be made up of many separate substances, and those from flowers are much more complicated than those from leaves – the former may have twelve to one hundred components, while some leaf essential oils may have only one!

Aromatherapists use them in their natural 'mixed' state, (when they are called terpenoids, because terpenes are present in the greatest quantity).

A chemist can break down the oil into its separate components of terpenes, esters, ketones etc., of which it is composed, and extract the part they want to use; for example, thymol is taken from thyme essential oil, and menthol is taken from peppermint essential oil. We are familiar with both these substances in present day medicine, but probably did not realize that they were from the actual essential oil produced from a plant.

Note: In general the more an essential oil is interfered with chemically or physically the more its therapeutic powers are reduced.

The strength at which an essential oil is used is very

important to remember, because some, if applied or taken in excess, or if too strong, have the reverse effect to that which is desired. For example, a low concentration of peppermint oil applied to an itchy skin will relieve the irritation; a strong concentration will aggravate the condition.

Similarly, digitalis, which is the essential oil of foxglove, is poisonous in high concentrations, but used carefully in medicine, it is very effective in relieving heart conditions.

It can be seen therefore that, when mixing oils for use in aromatherapy as well as in medicine, it is very important to use the correct concentration of essential oil, and also to realize that with many oils it does not necessarily follow that the more we use the better will be the result!

The high rate of evaporation of essential oils was mentioned earlier, and this is an important point to consider when mixing a well-balanced product. This volatility rate varies in different oils, and most essences fall into one of the following three classifications:

top notes	– the fastest acting, the quickest to evaporate, the most stimulating and uplifting to mind and body.
middle notes	– moderately volatile, primarily affect the functions of the body e.g., digestion, menstruation and the general metabolism of the body.
base notes	– slower to evaporate (if mixed with top note oil, it can help to 'hold back' the volatility of that oil), the most sedating and relaxing.

How Essential Oils are Obtained

Before distillation was invented, essential oils were extracted from the plants by hand expression, enfleurage and maceration.

Hand expression was confined to the citrus family, and the rinds were literally squeezed by hand until the oil glands or globules burst. The oil was collected in a sponge, which was squeezed into a container when saturated. This method is still used, but mostly by machines instead of hands.

Enfleurage was the method used for extracting essential oil from flowers, and is begun by placing the chosen flower heads on a glass bed covered with purified fat. The essential oils were absorbed by fat, the flowers removed, a new covering of flower heads put on and so on, repeating the process until the fat was saturated with essential oil. The resultant compound was called a 'pomade' and was often used in this state as an ointment or perfume. Enfleurage is still used as a method of extraction, but is usually carried to its second stage, which is to dissolve the pomade in alcohol. Fat is insoluble in alcohol but essential oil readily dissolves in it. The resultant liquid is then carefully heated, and as the alcohol evaporates first, the pure essential oil is left in the container.

Maceration is similar to enfleurage and is a method by which one can still make essential oil at home in a ready diluted state. The flowers or leaves are crushed to rupture some of the oil glands or cells, then put into warm vegetable oil (or purified fat) and put in a warm place. The vegetable oil or fat absorbs the essential oil and the flowers are strained off. A fresh lot of flowers or leaves is put into the re-warmed 'carrier' base, and this process is repeated until the vegetable oil or fat is concentrated enough. If fat is used, the resultant pomade can be treated as in the second stage of enfleurage; if vegetable oil is used, the resultant liquid can be used as it is for massage treatments, or in the making of home-made herbal creams.

Some flowers now have their oil taken from them by **solvent extraction** . In simple terms, the flowers are covered with a solvent, (usually petrol ether) which extracts the essential oil. The solvent is then evaporated off, leaving the essential oil in the container. It is a little more complicated than that, but that is the basic principle involved.

The most modern method, and the method most used nowadays, is **steam distillation**. Avicenna, an eleventh century Arabian physician, is credited with the invention of distillation as a method of extracting essential oils from plants, and Arnaldo de Vilanova (a Spaniard) probably gave the first authentic written description of the process of distillation in the thirteenth century, and may even have introduced this art to Europe.

Figure 1 (which may remind us of school days in the lab!) shows clearly how steam distillation is carried out. It depends on the density of the oil extracted as to whether it will float above the water, or sink below it, after condensation. This method makes use of the high volatility rate of essential oils plus

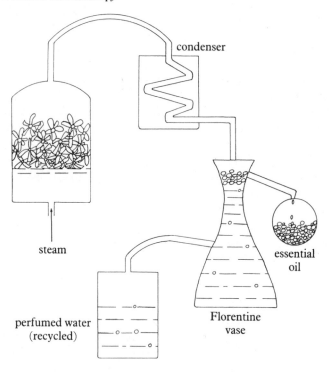

Figure 1. Steam distillation.

the fact that they are mainly insoluble in water. However, the same water going round and round the distillation plant does, after a time, become impregnated with the perfume or aroma of the plant being distilled, and is a useful by-product. Rose water and orange flower water are well-known examples.

The Purity of Essential Oils

From the account of the methods of extraction, the substances in which essential oils dissolve will be apparent. Mainly, they do not dissolve in water; they readily dissolve in alcohol; they dissolve in oil (vegetable or mineral) and they dissolve in fat. This information helps us to recognize a poor quality essential oil.

All essential oils are relatively expensive, though prices cover a wide range (depending mainly on percentage yield). If we see a low percentage yield oil, e.g., rose or jasmine, at a fairly low/medium price, it is probably not even a lower quality pure oil, but adulterated in some way, perhaps diluted in a solvent of some sort, or with added synthetic oils, the perfume of which can be a very good imitation of the real thing. So beware!

It is also difficult to compare prices of authentic essential oils, because one firm may import Chinese jasmine, which is a much lower price than jasmine from Morocco – at least three times the price! Sandalwood from Mysore (by far the best therapeutically) is at least twice the price of Australian Sandalwood, and so on.

As with most things the price is comparable with the quality, and the quality is definitely comparable with the results when essential oils are used for aromatherapy.

Synthetic substitutes are generally quite successful for cookery and perfumery, but it cannot be stressed enough that for the purpose of aromatherapy **only the best and purest** essential oils will give the desired effect.

By the way – essential oils are *not* greasy, though the name certainly suggests this. Most of them do not leave an oily mark on blotting paper, as would a drop of other oils we know , like corn oil, and their power of penetration through the skin and adjacent tissue is very great.

Storage of Essential Oils
Oils as we already know have a high evaporation rate; they are also sensitive to light, and care should be taken when using and storing them. Always replace the top after each application during the massage.

Because of their volatility they must be kept in tightly stoppered bottles; because they are sensitive to light, which can destroy them, they must be kept in dark bottles; because polythene tends to absorb essential oils they must be kept in glass or metal containers – in short, essential oils should be kept in air-tight, dark glass in a cool dark place for maximum shelf life.

For best results do not store ready mixed in a carrier oil for any length of time. Essential oils have a much longer life (up to eighteen to twenty-four months) if stored in their pure state.

3.

The Skin

The skin is the largest organ we have, covering and protecting the whole body, and it deserves to be taken care of. Any other organ which may be out of order and causing us discomfort is given immediate attention. But often the skin does not cause much discomfort when dry or cracked, or over oily, so we tend to think we are doing our best with it if we keep off soap and use skin care products for the prevailing condition.

In fact, a healthy skin reflects a healthy body and a blemished, flaking or irritable skin is often the result of some other part of us being out of order. We all know how our hair looks and feels when we are in low health; sometimes just a simple cold can make it lank and out of condition (even though it is dead matter according to Science!).

Owners of spotty or blemished skins often forget that what is *eaten* affects the skin (and hair) and if greasy or convenience foods form a large part of their diet, then the skin reflects this in its lack of glow, and perhaps spots or blackheads show themselves.

Stress can also affect the skin, causing it to be patchy and sensitive to certain products. Here it is necessary to get at the root cause, the stress or anxiety, and treat this in order to improve the skin.

Imperfect skin can also be due to hereditary causes. For instance, if you, or a relation, have, or have had, eczema, asthma or hay fever, it is possible for you to have a blemished skin, with dry patches. It is likely that you would presume yourself to be allergic to certain soaps or cosmetics, when in reality it is the eczema connection showing in your skin.

Similarly, if you suffer from psoriasis, you may think you are stuck with it except when you are using a cream from the doctor. Nothing completely cures psoriasis, except perhaps continual exposure to sunshine – difficult in England! – but solariums and sunbeds, if taken regularly can often keep psoriasis down to a minimum.

People who have dermatitis are often given a steroid cream to cure it. It does cure it, quickly, but there are side effects if the cream is used too often or for too long.

Quite a number of people, usually female, suffer from a super sensitive skin and find it very difficult to discover a brand of skincare which will not bring up an allergic reaction. Very often these ladies use a simple soap to avoid reactions, but of course, although it does the cleaning job well, it doesn't moisturize or feed or care for the skin in a way which will improve it.

Another sad story!

However, aromatherapy can help all these cases* and many more besides (including headaches and sinus problems!), by the use of good skin care products containing essential oils for their particular condition. And so, by spending *no extra time* on the daily skin care routine, many facial and skin problems can be dealt with automatically.

There is a range of skin care products which I have designed myself, mainly for the person who has a special problem with his or her skin. There are cleansers, toners, moisturizers, night cream, hand lotion, body lotion and masks – all designed to treat as well as to take care of the skin.* All creams and lotions are hypo-allergenic and are based on pure plant extracts. There is no lanolin in any of them, as lanolin (from sheep's wool) is responsible for a lot of allergies. There is no mineral oil in the moisturizers and night cream so maximum penetration is effected, to take care of the growing cells below the surface of the top skin. There is no animal product used and no perfume added. These too are other ingredients which can often be responsible for many allergic reactions.

So before we even start mentioning essential oils, the products are suitable for a very sensitive skin, which is important in itself.

Then we come to the interesting part. To the basic product different essential oils are added to help different types of skin; not just sensitive, dry, combination and oily, but eczema, dermatitis, sinus blockage, psoriasis, broken veins, stress, insomnia, persistent headaches, etc. By using these every day you can help to clear up your problem, yet do nothing more than a normal skin care routine! And in most cases it costs no more than many well-known brands.

*See Case Histories. Chap. 13.
*See Useful Addresses

For those who are not accustomed to using a skin care routine I am going to set out a programme for you to follow. Those of you who do not like cleansing creams or lotions because you like to rinse your face with water, will be very pleased to know that cleansers are now available, including my own, which are water soluble and can be rinsed off in the same way as soap if wished.

The Skin

The surface of our skin (the epidermis) is completely made up of dead, yes, dead, skin cells. In a baby and young child these are continually and quickly thrown off by the newer cells underneath, which in their turn are thrown off themselves. A child's skin is normally moist, rounded and smooth because of the speedy regeneration of new cells everywhere in the body, and equally speedy throwing off of dead ones. As we get older of course, the regeneration of new cells slows down (not just in the skin) and old dead cells are slower in being thrown off. This can be responsible, in part, for dry skin, and is certainly an aid in the acquiring of wrinkles, where the dead cells collect in the little furrows of the skin and our facial expressions push them into line formation.

Soap, although a fairly efficient cleanser, usually has an alkaline base, and for the elasticity of the skin to be preserved, alkaline substances are not good. This is because the skin is slightly acid (in order to kill bacteria which may invade the tissue) and using an alkaline cleanser removes this needed acidity. It is also very drying, hence oily skinned people think soap is good for them. Certainly oily skinned people stay younger-looking for longer, but often they pay for the privilege by having a spotty or open-pored skin in their late teens (due mainly to hormonal changes and also to incorrect diet).

Underneath the epidermis we have a layer of skin called the dermis. This is alive, and contains all the blood vessels, nerve endings, oil and sweat glands. Here, new skin cells are made and pushed upwards, and as they reach the epidermis they flatten, die off and are eventually thrown off the skin surface.

The skin is waterproof and only the epidermis gets wet and needs to be dried off. Because of this quality, not many substances can penetrate the skin – in fact many doctors pooh-pooh skin creams as anything but surface protectors. With lotions containing mineral oil we know this to be true – they give the effect of moisturizing the skin because they *do* keep the *surface* moist. But we will learn in a later chapter that mineral oil does not penetrate the skin too well, therefore no improvement can be given to the living cells underneath the top skin – we are just keeping the top skin temporarily moist.

Creams containing lanolin are similar in their non-effectiveness as skin regenerators. Lanolin particles are usually too large to penetrate the skin, as anyone who uses a night cream rich in lanolin will know – not only does the face look greasy, but the cream penetrates the pillow more than the face. Vegetable oil based creams and lotions, on the other hand, are able to have slight penetration into the skin.

Essential oils, as we have seen, are *highly* penetrative and can reach the small blood capillaries in the dermis, from whence they are carried in the blood to actually do something useful. At the same time, if the *right* oils are added, the skin can be rejuvenated, i.e., better quality skin cells are made, because they are fed with the right ingredients; so they look smoother and feel softer and less dry or less oily, (as the case may be) as they reach the skin surface and die off.

Opening onto the skin are two special types of gland; the sweat glands and the sebaceous or oil glands. The latter produce a natural oil called sebum, which comes onto the skin surface via the hair follicle. So where there are no hairs at all, there is no oil, i.e., palms of hands, soles of feet, eye area.

The job of sebum is to lubricate the skin and preserve its elasticity.

The sweat glands produce a watery, yet slightly oily, liquid we call perspiration, which escapes onto the skin surface via pore openings. The palms of the hands have the most sweat glands, though there are many present in the soles of the feet, the armpits and on the forehead and nose too.

Sweat glands eliminate body waste and toxins and also provide the body's own cooling system, so when we are hot, through exerting ourselves, these glands send out extra moisture to help cool the body down. Normally, to maintain body temperature, we don't notice our sweat glands working but in wind, sun and central heating especially, this normal amount of moisture produced evaporates too quickly, leaving the skin drier than it should be. This is why it is essential to use a moisturizer daily to help to counteract this loss.

The sweat and oil glands work *together* to keep the surface of the skin supple and balanced. If one type of gland is over- or under-productive, then this shows itself in an oily or dry skin type.

Using the correct moisturizer for the skin type helps to balance this and keep the skin supple. Even people with over-productive oil glands need a moisturizer to replace the *moisture* lost, which is causing the oil to predominate. *But* it must then be a moisturizer which contains a minimal amount of oil, but is mainly water in a light emulsion.

Every time the face and neck are washed, a moisturizer should be applied, because all the natural oil and moisture on the skin surface has been washed off and to protect the skin a moisture lotion or moisture cream should be used on face and neck afterwards.

This does three things for us:

i.   Counteracts unnatural moisture loss.
ii. Keeps oil and moisture content of skin balanced.
iii. Protects pore openings from dirt and make-up, which can clog them and cause blackheads and spots.

You can see now that everyone needs a moisturizer (even men should use one!) but not everyone needs a night cream. A night cream lubricates the skin and (provided a good vegetable based one is used) also feeds the growing cells in the dermis, ensuring improvement in the elasticity. Oily skinned people do not generally need a night cream until they feel their skin is beginning to dry out on the cheek area, then one should be used around the eyes, (never use a lanolin based cream around the eyes), on the cheeks and all over the neck area. Remember, there are not any oil glands on the eyes and very few on the neck, so don't neglect the areas that need feeding just because you have a very oily strip down the centre of your face.

A night cream does two important things:

i.   Replaces oil where glands are not functioning properly, or are slowing down due to getting older.
ii. Keeps skin well lubricated and so minimizes the risk of early wrinkles due to loss of skin elasticity.

Two other areas which need feeding as we get older, because the pores are not producing so much moisture, are our hands and feet. Use of a body lotion after each shower or bath can take care of dry feet, legs and hands, and hand lotion, applied every time the hands are washed, helps to keep them supple and moist, and there is one which is particularly good for chapped hands.

Special areas need treatment with masks:

Very oily skin down centre of face.
Very dry skin on face and neck.
Fine wrinkle lines at sides of eyes and mouth, forehead and upper lip.
Sallow skin, lacking in tone and colour.
Dry backs of heels, elbows and knees and dry hands.

Dry and sallow areas need a feeding mask or a mask which will activate the blood circulation, thus bringing nutrients to the area. Very oily areas need a mask which will clean out pores and oil glands.

Wrinkle lines need a mask to clean out dead skin cells from furrows (use a moisturizer immediately afterwards).

Sensitive skins should never need a treatment mask, but natural yogurt with liquidized cucumber will soothe and freshen any type of skin, including the sensitive one.

Skin Care Routine

The aim of skin care is to encourage all types of skin to become normal through the correct use of the correct skin care products, and combination skins should use the cleanser and moisturizer to suit the area which is the greatest problem. Those with oily panels should use a mask to rectify, and a cleanser and moisturizer to suit the cheek area.

Caring for the skin takes no longer than washing with soap and water. The only additional few seconds is the use of a toner and moisturizer.

Every night:
Cleanse face and neck thoroughly – rinse off.
Apply toner on cotton wool.
Put night cream (or moisturizer when you don't need night cream) on face, neck and eyes* (or moisture lotion if very oily).
Eye creams and gels without lanolin or mineral oil can be used on any skin type.
Every morning:
Wipe face, neck and eyes with toner on cotton wool. (Not necessary to cleanse again unless you want to.)
Apply moisturizer to face, neck and eyes* then make-up if worn.
*Not on eyes if cream is lanolin based.

If at any time after this you want to wear make-up you need to re-moisturize immediately before applying it, or cleanse, tone and moisturize first if more than four hours later.

Once a week (twice for an oily panel) a treatment mask should be used if it is needed. People with a normal skin only need a mask every now and again, except for the yogurt and cucumber type, which can be used as often as you wish.

It is very important that you use a spatula with jars of cream. Not only is it economical, but also it prevents your putting in any bacteria which may be under your nails and may multiply in the cream.

The following table should be of help, and if you have a combination skin use the cleanser and moisturizer to suit the cheek area, and use a mask for open pores and blackheads on the oily panel once or twice a week.

	Sensitive	Oily	Normal	Dry
Cleansing Cream	★		★	★
Cleansing Milk	★	★	★	
Alcohol-free Toning Lotion	★	★	★	★
Lanolin+mineral oil-free Moisture Lotion	★	★	★	
Lanolin+mineral oil-free Moisture Cream	★		★	★
Lanolin+mineral oil-free Night Cream	★	★	★	★
Lanolin+mineral oil-free Eye Creams and Gels	★	★	★	★
Mask for open pores and blackheads		★	★	★
Feeding Mask	★	★	★	★
Mask for stimulating the blood circulation		★	★	★
Yogurt and Cucumber	★	★	★	★

BASIC SKIN CARE PROCEDURE

Cleansing

PRODUCT	METHOD	ACTION
Cleansing Creams (use a spatula) Effectively cleanse normal or dry skin. Very dry skins should always use a cream.	1. Small amount on finger tips; place fingers of both hands together. 2. Using both hands massage cream in upward and outward circles over neck and face. 3. Eye circles should start on upper lid at nose and come to temple, returning to nose underneath the eye. (One continuous circle). 4. Rinse off with water, or wipe off with damp cotton wool.	1. Removes stale make-up from skin surface. 2. Removes accumulated skin secretions. 3. Removes dust and dirt. (Excellent for make-up round the eyes for any skin-type). 4. Helps to normalize a dry skin.
Cleansing Milks These have the same properties as cleansing cream, but in the form of a lotion, which is suitable for any skin which is not very dry.	As for cleansing creams	1. Removes stale make-up from skin surface. 2. Removes accumulated skin secretions. 3. Removes dust and dirt. 4. Helps to normalize an oily skin.

PRODUCT	METHOD	ACTION
Alcohol-free Toning Lotions A natural toner to freshen, tone and re-vitalize the skin. Suitable for all skin types, even the most sensitive, as it is non-drying	1. Moisten cotton wool with toner (hold on bottle and tip up twice for correct amount.) 2. Wipe gently over face and neck, upwards and outwards.	1. Refreshes and cools skin. 2. Tones facial muscles. 3. Removes any remaining traces of cleanser plus make-up or dirt. 4. Can be used as a cleanser where make-up has not been worn, i.e., first thing in the morning.

Conditioning

PRODUCT	METHOD	ACTION
Masks for open pores & blackheads (use a spatula)	1. Small amount on back of hand. 2. Massage into the skin in small circles for 2 to 3 minutes, wherever the problem is, keeping it moist. (Dip finger in water if necessary). 3. Do not use *under* eyes but on corners of eyes and along upper lip to help prevent premature wrinkling. 4. Rinse off with warm water and pat dry. 5. Follow with moisture lotion or cream.	1. Normalizes an oily skin. 2. Stimulates and refreshes. 3. Gentle abrasive action lifts out dead skin cells lying in valleys of skin, thus making wrinkle-lines less obvious. 4. Helps remove blackheads. 5. Helps spots (unless medical in origin). 6. Refines open pores. 7. Deep cleanses a greasy skin. 8. Smooths rough skin (heels, elbows, etc.)

PRODUCT	METHOD	ACTION
Feeding Masks (use a spatula) Mixed with equal part of natural yogurt makes a superb soothing and cooling mask.	1. Take about a teaspoonful and spread *quickly* and evenly over the skin of face and neck (even under the eyes). Do not rub in. 2. Leave for the time stated. 3. Rinse off with warm water and pat dry. 4. Follow with moisture lotion or cream.	1. Normalizes a dry skin. 2. Refreshes and smooths. 3. Gently stimulates circulation. 4. Softens dead skin cells on surface which are removed with mask. 5. Refines pores. 6. Smooths and softens hands.
Masks to promote blood circulation. (Use a spatula). Effective treatment mask for skin improvement but must be used with care. Can be mixed with natural yogurt on a sensitive skin.	1. As in 1 above - Feeding Masks. 2. Sensitive skin — leave for *1 minute only* on first treatment, increasing to 3 minutes after 4 to 5 treatments. Sallow, dull skin—leave for 15 to 20 minutes. (Adjust for skin types in between.) 3. and 4. as above.	1. Normalizes a sensitive skin. 2. Activates blood circulation to promote healthy skin. 3. Acts as mild skin peeling, removing dead skin cells from surface. 4. Refines pores. 5. Good feeding mask for hands and feet.

Note: Always remove *any* mask immediately if prickling sensation occurs before the required time.

Protecting

PRODUCT	METHOD	ACTION
Moisture Lotions (without lanolin or mineral oil) A light lotion to give an oily or normal skin the right amount of moisture needed to keep the skin supple. Non-greasy, therefore excellent for keeping eyelids well moistened and supple.	1. Small amount on tips of fingers; place fingers of both hands together. 2. 'Run' over face *and neck* with tips of fingers. 3. Blend lotion into face and neck with outward and upward movements. 4. Do not forget to include the eyelids! These *need* moisture protection.	1. Helps to normalize an oily skin. 2. Keeps skin's natural moisture balance correct, by replacing moisture lost through sweat glands. 3. Forms a barrier to help prevent dust, dirt and make-up going into pores.
Moisture Creams (without lanolin or mineral oil.) (use a spatula) A day cream to give a normal to dry skin the right amount of moisture to keep the skin supple and free from flaking.	As in Moisture Lotions. Do not forget eyes and neck.	1. Helps to normalize a dry skin. 2. and 3. as in Moisture Lotions. 4. Helps to maintain a higher level of moisture in the skin.

Preserving

PRODUCT	METHOD	ACTION
Night Creams (without lanolin) (Use a spatula). Specially formulated to keep a high degree of moisture in the skin and aid in the retardation of ageing. Suitable for all skin types, because they should be completely non-greasy.	As in Moisture Lotions and do not forget eyes and neck. *Note:* Oily skins should use once a week. Dry skins should use every night.	1. Softens and beautifies skin. 2. Keeps wrinkles at bay. 3. Helps to preserve natural elasticity of skin.
Eye Creams and Gels. (without lanolin) (Use a spatula) Specially made for the extra sensitive skin around the eyes, they will help to prevent wrinkles and keep skin supple.	1. Take a very small amount onto ring fingers only. 2. Circle round eyes from nose to temple on upper lid and back to nose under eye. Continue circling. 3. Can also be used on upper lip where fine vertical lines start to form.	1. Keeps skin around eyes soft and supple. 2. Softens existing lines. 3. Helps prevent new lines forming.

4.

Yin, Yang and Shiatsu

Shiatsu is a massage originating from the East and is sometimes referred to as 'acupuncture without needles', or 'acupressure'. It is an energy flow massage, and in order to use it successfully the whole mind must be concentrated on the client.

To understand Shiatsu (finger pressure) massage more thoroughly it is necessary to study the meaning of Yin and Yang principles.

In the East all natural forces are divided into two categories; passive (or negative) forces and active (or positive) forces called Yin and Yang respectively. (Physical forces are divided into five categories – wood, fire, water, earth and metal.)

Yin and Yang always have a balancing interplay, both in nature and in the human personality. Nature balances itself, but when the human body is out of order in any way, the Yin Yang balance is upset, and can be helped by someone understanding these forces. To make it a little clearer, here are a few Yin and Yang characteristics:

Yin	Yang
negative	positive
passive	active
'female'	'male'
dark	light
earth	heaven
empty	full

Just as these Yin and Yang characteristics complement one another, so does the list below show their interplay and harmony in nature and human beings. For balance:

rain needs sunshine to follow it
a storm will be followed by calm
a thirsty person drinks to satisfy his thirst
after a stimulating sport the body must relax
a depressed person needs to be uplifted
a highly strung person needs to be calmed

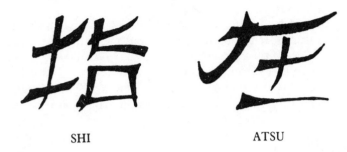

SHI   ATSU

In the human body there are invisible lines along which the body energy flows. They are called meridian lines and connect with the organs in the body. These organs (and their meridian lines) complement one another, and so are called either Yin meridians or Yang meridians.

Yang meridians all flow down the body from head to foot, including the arms when held above the head (i.e., from fingers to shoulders).

Yin Meridians
heart (inside arm)
heart constrictor (inside arm)
lung (inside arm)
spleen (front of body)
liver (front of body)
kidney (front of body)

Yang Meridians
small intestine (outside arm)
triple heater (outside arm)
large intestine (outside arm)
bladder (back of body)
gall-bladder (side of body)
stomach (front of body and side of leg)

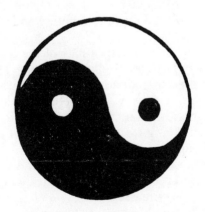

Yin meridians all flow up the body from feet to head, including the arms when held above the head (i.e., from shoulders to fingers).

There are points along these lines which connect to various parts of our systems, both physical and mental, and pressure put on these points correctly can keep the body in good general health or relieve symptoms already there.

People also come into a general Yin or Yang category. Although different aspects of each person may be Yin or Yang, and though these are changing all the time, basically a person follows most of the time a Yin-type or a Yang-type pattern of behaviour.

Yin	**Yang**
slender	well made
weak	strong
listless	active

This is rather important to remember, because if we diagnose someone as Yin, all the Shiatsu massage on that person must be done in the direction of the meridian flow; i.e., up the Yin meridians and down the Yang meridians.

Also the pressure applied is different for each type, though for both it should be applied only as the client is breathing *out*.

Yin	**Yang**
slow gentle pressure	quick strong pressure
slow release	quick release
with meridian flow	*against* meridian flow

Shiatsu pressure points are more difficult to find than the reflex points in reflexology, and a lot of practice and experience is needed in order to have maximum ability and give maximum benefits.

In my aromatherapy massage many of the Shiatsu pressure points are covered automatically during the treatment, but these may be pressed individually as a separate treatment, covering only those points where relief is actually needed, and following the meridian line in the correct direction for the particular person being treated, depending on whether he or she is Yin or Yang.

All this sounds very confusing – indeed, it *is* confusing – and one needs to visit an experienced Shiatsu therapist to benefit fully from this type of massage.

However, it is possible for you to carry out *some* Shiatsu, combined with effleurage, so long as the principles of Yin and Yang are fully understood, further reading is done on the meridian lines, and there is complete empathy or feeling between the giver and the receiver of the massage.

I will list the points most commonly required, including those covered by the massage given, in the chapter on Aromatherapy Massage Techniques.

Before pressing shiatsu pressure points (such a point is called a tsubo) it is best to stroke the meridian line first gently with the thumbs in the right direction, depending on whether the client is Yin or Yang, then do the pressures in numerical order, low to high or high to low, depending again on the client's Yin or Yang tendencies. If this is too complicated, the pressures will still be reasonably effective done on their own provided the correct type of pressure is used, and the client's Yin or Yang state is taken into consideration for these.

To enable all the information on identifying pressure points to be tabulated more easily across the page it is necessary to abbreviate the names of the meridian lines as follows:

Yang (see *Figure 2.*)

bladder meridian –	b – off centre back and legs
gall-bladder meridian –	gb – side of body and legs
governing vessel –	gv – centre back and head
stomach meridian –	st – side front and legs
liver meridian –	lv – side front and legs
large intestine meridian –	li – outside arm

Yin (see *Figure 3.*)

kidney meridian –	k – off centre front and legs
spleen meridian –	sp – side front and legs
lung meridian –	l – inside arm
heart meridian –	h – inside arm
heart constrictor meridian –	hc – inside arm
conception vessel –	cv – centre front

All the meridian lines and all the pressure points in the body are not mentioned in this book; just a useful selection.

The names of the vertebrae are also abbreviated, i.e.,

C = Cervical (neck area)
T = Thoracic (shoulder blade area)
L = Lumbar (back area)
S = Sacrum (base of spinal column.)

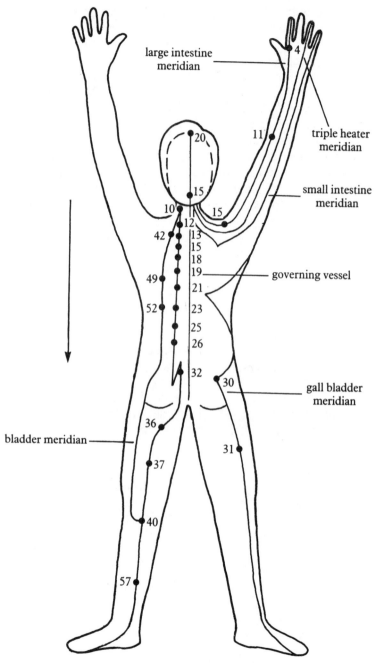

Figure 2. Yang meridians.

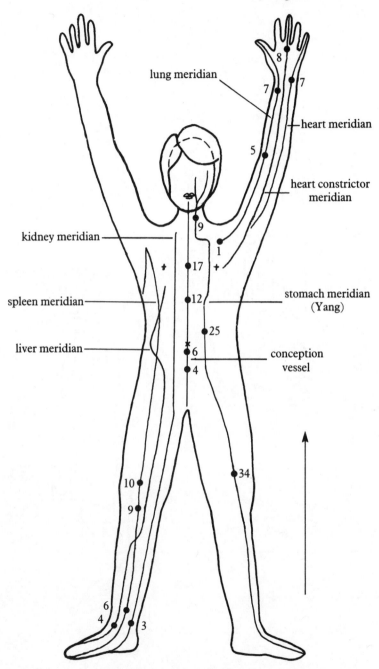

Figure 3. Yin meridians.

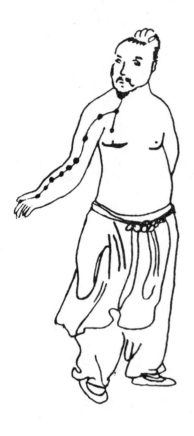

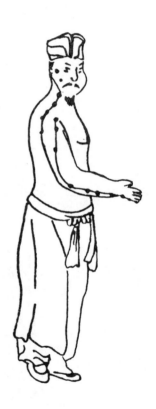

PRESSURE POINT IDENTIFICATION TABLE

P.Point	Disorder	Position	Name
Back			
(a)b 10	headache; nasal conditions	C1—2 2½cm from spine centre	Ten Chu—pillar of heaven
(b)b 12	breathing problems	T2—3 2½cm from spine centre	Fu Mon—gate of wind
(c)b 13	chest conditions	T3—4 2½cm from spine centre	Hai Yu—lung associated point
(d)b 42	neck and shoulder pains	T3—4 7½cm from spine centre	Haku Ko
(e)b 15	irritability; weak heart	T5—6 2½cm from spine centre	Shin Yu—heart associated point
(f)b 18	liver conditions; sea sickness	T9—10 2½cm from spine centre	Kan Yu—liver associated point
(g)b 19	gall-bladder conditions	T10—11 2½cm from spine centre	Tan Yu—gall-bladder associated point
(h)b 49	stomach ache; nervous tension	T11—12 7½cm from spine centre	I Sha
(i)b 21	stomach problems	T12—L1 2½cm from spine centre	I Yu—stomach associated point
(j)b 23	revitalization; kidney conditions	L2—3 2½cm from spine centre	Jin Yu—kidney associated point
(k)b 52	lower backache; kidney conditions; lack of energy	L2—3 7½cm from spine centre	Shi Shitsu—chamber of spirits
(l)b 25	constipation	L4—5 2½cm from spine centre	Dai Cho Yu—large intestine associated point
(m)b 26	digestion; sexual conditions	L5—S1 2½cm from spine centre	Kan Gen Yu
(n)b 32	menstrual irregularities	second groove in sacrum	Gi Ryo—second hole
Legs (back)			
(a)b 36	sciatica: lower backache	centre top thigh, buttock base	Sho Fu
(b)b 37	sciatica; tired legs	mid-back thigh, 15cm below buttock crease	I Mon

P.Point	Disorder	Position	Name
Legs (back) continued			
(c)b 40	lower backache; calf cramp	centre back of knee	I Chu
(d)b 57	sciatica; tired legs; cramp	centre gastrocnemius (calf) muscle at its insertion*	Shyo Zan—in the mountain
(e)gb 30	sciatica; lower backache	indentation on side of buttock	Kan Chyo
(f)gb 31	poor leg circulation	client's middle finger tip when hand down by side	Fu Shi—market of wind
Legs (front)			
(a)st 34	stomach pains; arthritis in knee	5cm above knee cap and slightly toward outside of leg (find with knee bent)	Rio Kyu—on the hill
(b)k 3	kidney conditions	between inside ankle bone and Achilles tendon	Tai Kei—great groove
(c)sp 6	insomnia; overweight; menstrual pain; digestive problems	client's little finger on top of inside ankle bone—behind shin and level with index finger	San Yin Ko—meeting point of the 3 Yin leg meridians
(d)sp 9	pain in knee	top of shin bone on inside leg	Yin Ryo Sen—Yin mountain pond
(e)sp 10	nerve rash; itching; menstrual pain	indentation on inside leg 5cm diagonally up from knee cap	Ketsu Kai—ocean of blood
(f)lv 4	arthritis in ankle	just past ankle bone towards top of foot	Chu Ho

* about half way between the knee and heel where that muscle begins.

P.Point	Disorder	Position	Name
Scalp			
(a)gb 20	common cold; headache	2½cm behind mastoid process	Fu Chi—pond of wind
(b)b 10	headache; nasal obstruction	base of occipitalis, 2½cm from centre and 2½cm down	Ten Chu—pillar of heaven
(c)gv 15	headaches; colds	C1—2 centre spine	A Mon—gate of fool
(d)gv 20	headache	centre top of head	Hya Kue—one hundred meetings
(e)gv 23	headache; nasal problems	client's middle finger tip when wrist on nose	Jo Sei—upper star
Face			
(a)st 1	tension; tired vision	along nasal bone under eye centre	Sho Kyu
(b)st 3	sinus; nasal congestion; facial tension	4cm below stomach 1 on a level with the nose base	Kyo Sho
(c)st 4	facial tension; general tension	mouth corners	Chi So
(d)st 6	toothache	2½cm in front of ear lobe base	Kyo Shya
(e)cv(end)	facial and mouth tension	between lower lip and chin	
(f)b 1	headache; tired eyes	inside corner of eye	Sei Mei—bright light
(g)gb 1	eye problems; headache	hollow 2½cm from outside eye corner	Do Shi Ryo
(h)gb 2	ringing in the ears	hollow directly in front of and above ear lobe	Cho E—hearing point
	headaches; nasal obstruction	between eyebrows	In Do
	headaches; swollen eyes; dizziness .	just behind hair line and 2½cm diagonally up from gb 1	Tai Yo

P.Point	Disorder	Position	Name
Arms			
(a)li 4	general health; toothache	in between thumb and index finger	Go Kuku—meeting mountains
(b)li 11	any arm problems	just below crease made when elbow is bent	Kyoku Chi—lake of energy
(c)li 15	shoulder joint pains; frozen shoulder	on indentation just past shoulder bone on top of shoulder	Ken Gu—corner of shoulder
(d)l 5	cough; painful breathing	just above li 11, and below tendon	Shoku Taku—in the groove
(e)l 7	congestion; headaches	in direct line with thumb about 2½cm past wrist	Retsu Ketsu
(f)h 7	insomnia; irritability	just above and diagonally from outside wrist bone	Shin Mon—gate of god
(g)hc 8	exhaustion	between middle and ring fingers when fingers are bent to touch palm	Ro Kyu—palace of anxiety
Abdomen			
(a)cv 4	frigidity; menstrual problems	7½cm below the navel	Kan Gen—gate of origin
(b)cv 6	stomach ache; constipation; diarrhoea	4cm below the navel	Ki Kai—ocean of energy
		The area covering the above pressure points is called . . .	Tan Den
(c)cv 12	nausea, vomiting	centre abdomen, 10cm above navel	Chu Kan—midway
(d)st 25	stomach pains; diarrhoea	5cm laterally from navel	Ten Su

5.

Reflexology

Reflexology cannot easily be defined simply from its name, as can many other therapies, e.g., psychology, aromatherapy, etc. It may partly be due to this that reflexology is also known by other more easily explained terms, such as 'zone therapy', 'compression massage' and 'press point therapy'.

In our western medical books nine bodily systems are known. They can be found in the body, and the way in which they function can be logically worked out and proven. But the western world is just beginning to accept that less easily explained 'systems' do exist in the human body, systems which, in the East, have been used for hundreds of years to diagnose and to treat the nine known systems and their related organs. The 'meridian lines system' in acupuncture and acupressure is one example and the 'zones system' in press point therapy or reflexology is another. Reflexology is one of the few therapies which brings relief through remote application.

Many books have been written on reflexology and as this book is mainly about aromatherapy it is not possible to spend too much time on the subject. However, the following points make a good summary of its uses:

Reflexology:
  (a) is a speedy and accurate method of diagnosis
  (b) is a treatment of disorders by natural means
  (c) is useful as a preventative for disease
  (d) relaxes the whole body and mind, and is therefore invaluable as a release from tension – the world's most popular 'disease' at this time

In a way 'reflexology' is a slightly misleading term and in order for it to be understood more easily it is necessary to explain what it is *not*!

Our Nervous System

From the nervous systems in our body spring voluntary and involuntary reactions to specific conditions.

The job of the nervous system is to convey information from the world outside and conditions inside our body to the brain, and also to transmit instructions from the brain to all parts of our body. (See *Figure 4*.)

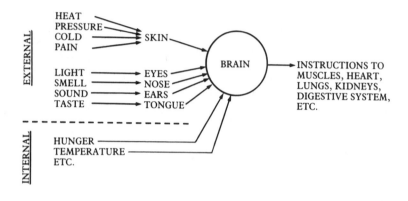

Figure 4

A voluntary reaction is when we make a conscious decision to do something. Perhaps there is a pen lying on the table; our eyes pick up the light reflections and the information is transmitted to the brain; the brain decides to pick up the pen and sends the message to the appropriate muscles of the arm and hand.

An involuntary reaction occurs, for example, if we touch a

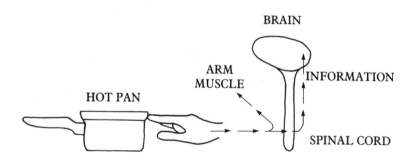

Figure 5

hot pan. The heat sensors in the skin send an urgent warning message which, in this emergency situation, is dealt with by the spinal cord and a signal goes from here to the muscles of the arm to remove the hand from danger. At the same time a message goes up to the brain, which becomes aware of what is going on and prepares the body for further action. An involuntary reaction is also known as a reflex action. (See *Figure 5*.)

There are other reflex actions which occur in the autonomic – (involuntary or automatic) nervous system and as the name suggests these are carried out without our having any conscious knowledge about them, e.g., the heart continues beating without our telling it to all the time; similarly our digestive system keeps on working without direct orders continually from our conscious brain (which is very fortunate for us!).

The autonomic nervous system is characterized by a chain of little energy centres containing masses of nerve cells and there are several main groups of these in the body which are called plexuses. The coeliac (or solar) plexus is the largest and most 'responsive' plexus to consciousness, and it has a unique importance in that it is the centre of feelings and emotions. It is from here, under certain conditions, that quite pronounced and definite physical sensations of discomfort may be initiated.

The reflexes mentioned above are well understood in western society and can be found in medical textbooks. However, the reflexes which occur in reflexology are not the same as those within the nervous system. Not much is known medically about them – it is still very much an art and not a science – and as with meridian lines they do not show on an X-ray or on dissection. All that is known is that the system works; reflexology is in widespread use in many parts of the world and can be used in diagnosis as well as treatment. Experience has also shown that unlike nerves, these energy reflexes do not cross over the spinal column, and react *without* going through the spinal connector nerves, following instead the body's zone lines. For example, the eye reflex in the left foot will react from the *left* eye and not in the right as might be expected from study of the central nervous system. Organs which are in the same zone are often related and the related reflex (as well as the affected reflex) may show a blockage, e.g., eyes and kidneys are in the same zone.

Hence the nearest we can get to a definition of reflexology is that it is an ancient eastern technique which makes use of somewhat mysterious connecting pathways or energy flow lines in the body. (See *Figure 6*.)

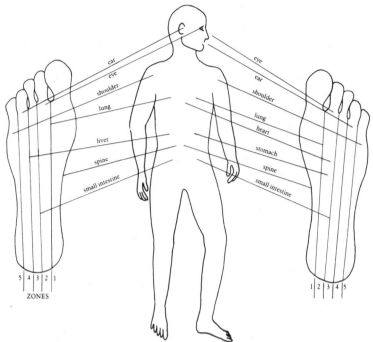

Figure 6. General relationship of body part to foot area.

What Reflexology is and How it can Help You

When pressure is applied where these lines come to the surface, this brings about relaxation and is a great help in normalizing body conditions. These points are easiest to find in the feet, though they are to be found in other extremities of the body, i.e., hands and ears. It must be mentioned here that these points can only indicate the probable organs where there may be some disorder. It does not indicate the cause of the disorder, only that some disorder is there.

Reflexology is not a cure, though in the hands of an experienced practitioner it can effect a cure. Neither is it intended to provide a substitute for medical diagnoses or treatment. It is, however, extremely helpful and is without any of the side-effects which normally accompany conventional drugs and medicine. Success depends on the ability to give accurate massage on the reflexes. Each organ and muscle in the body is connected without crossing the spinal column by an energy pathway to a point in the foot, hand, ear, etc. (See *Figure 7*.)

The most fascinating thing about these reflex points, is that

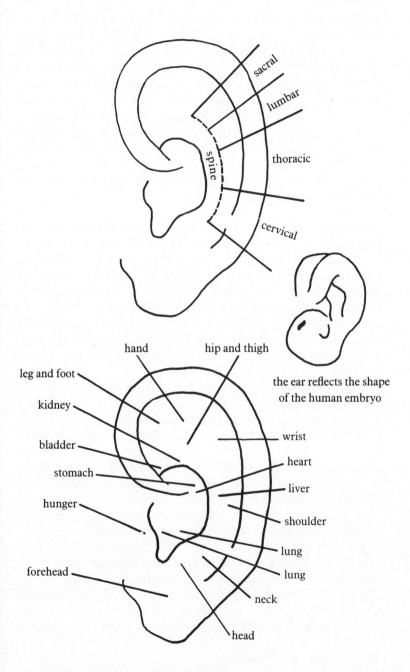

Figure 7. Acupressure areas of the ear.

they come to the surface in exactly the same position as they are found in the body, and are mostly found on the soles of the feet. If you imagine that with the feet close together, the big toes are the head, the balls of the feet are the shoulders and down the centre is the spine – the curve of each foot here is even identical to the side view of a person's back. The foot even narrows around the waist area. Thus, all organs found above the waist in the body are found above the waist of the foot, those positioned below are found below. So it can be seen that a sound knowledge of anatomy is of great help in reflexology and, indeed, the best reflexologists would be those with a medical or nursing background.

If there is a malfunction for any reason in the blood circulation, which in turn affects the organs nearest to this malfunction, a blockage occurs in the energy pathway and crystalline deposits form at the reflex point representing the organ where the disorder is showing itself. It is not really known whether these deposits are in the blood circulation at the changeover from arteries to veins, or at the nerve endings. But they can definitely be felt when they are present, and equally definitely can be broken down by correct pressure massage, bringing about relaxation plus a relief from the symptoms being suffered.

The principle of good health is one of balance, when all bodily systems are behaving as nature intended, complementing one another to give the body this balance, or good health. The human body, apart from its more mysterious attributes, like the ability to think, is an intricate machine in which the blood acts like oil; therefore it is of prime importance to the working of that machine that the blood circulation flows unimpeded throughout the body.

If there is congestion in the body the circulation is poor. If the circulation is upset by tension or stress then illness can occur, as the organs do not receive enough blood. (See *Figure 8*.) Each cell is contracting and relaxing every moment, and when distress occurs this cannot be as regulated as it should be, and the healthy circulation is interfered with, resulting eventually in unhealthy organs. Every organ and every part of the body *needs* a correct flow of blood in order to be completely healthy.

Reflexology as a Diagnosis
All practising aromatherapists use reflexology for diagnostic purposes only; those who want to practise reflexology as a

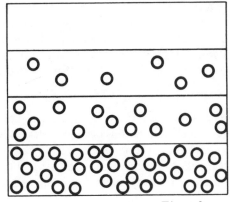

Good health — full blood supply

1. Failing Circulation

2. Unhealthy tissue

3. Disease

Figure 8.

treatment in its own right have to do further training. However, as I have explained in the chapter on Aromatherapy Massage, many people have a natural talent for some practical subjects and, for those, I am explaining the method of treatment in full.

When reflexology is used as a diagnostic check on someone, the reflex points are pressed only long enough to tell whether or not there is a disorder present, and all the bodily systems are covered in turn. The treatment which follows is then concentrated only on the systems which showed blockage, and the pressure applied varies slightly in duration as well as intensity.

How to Recognize a Blockage

The blockage at a reflex point is always felt by someone when pressure is correctly applied. The feeling varies from a strange unpleasant feeling to a sharp knife-like pain or a rippling as though lead shot was under the skin. This latter is the only reaction the operator can feel and for the other two he has to rely on the reactions of the person. Because of this, the operator's eyes should carefully watch the person's *face*, as well as the feet being worked on. Three or four minutes on a troubled reflex is usually enough at one treatment for anyone.

Reflexology stimulates the blood circulation and all the systems in the body, so do not treat anyone who

1. has just finished a meal or is needing food!
2. is at the beginning of a heavy period
3. is under heavy sedation or on a lot of tablets (except gently here, as usually this type of person *needs* reflexology).

The first time a person is given reflexology the pain felt where there is a blockage may be quite severe. This does not necessarily indicate a severe disorder and can sometimes be caused by tension in that person. It is a good idea, therefore, to commence all treatments, especially the first, by a series of preliminary massage movements to induce a relaxed conditon. The solar plexus should also be gently massaged for the same reason.

Related Areas and Reflexes

Firstly, it must be clearly understood that as organs in the body are often positioned over one another, or overlapping in some way, so therefore are the reflexes that represent them. This means that when one gets a reaction, say, on the stomach reflex, it may be the pancreas which has the problem; similarly part of the left lung overlaps the heart, etc. Thus it can be seen that one has to be careful when *asking* questions about a reaction, and even more careful when replying to the *person's* questions, so as not to frighten him or her unnecessarily. Should the operator suspect there is something serious present, he should refer that person to a doctor. Otherwise it is better to talk about general areas rather than specific points, and not to state exactly what one thinks has been found. Reflex therapy on the whole tender area can still be given, with beneficial results, even if one cannot pinpoint the exact area requiring treatment.

Reflexes are also related to one another. If there is a definite disorder in the stomach area all the points in the digestive system should be massaged; similarly if the kidney area shows a disorder, all organs connected with excretion should be massaged.

The Importance of Relaxation

Always make certain that the person being treated is sitting comfortably or lying down as it is essential for him to be as relaxed as possible. The blood circulation – the key to all bodily functions – flows correctly only in a relaxed body. As I said before, it is when tension is present in an area that the blood cannot flow through evenly, toxins are not removed fast enough and a disorder sets itself up.

The operator should also be relaxed and comfortable, and must give complete concentration to what he or she is doing, with no other thoughts in his mind.

The diagnosis and massage must never be automatic but, as in all contact treatments like aromatherapy and shiatsu, there must be totaly empathy between operator and recipient, and when this exists the energy flow goes from one to the other, making the benefits more satisfying and lasting.

Before commencing work on the actual reflex points it is a great help to have the person being treated breathing in a slow, relaxed manner. Show him how to take deep breaths, filling his lungs and slowly exhaling; breathe with him until a comfortable rhythm is established. Then, with the person continuing with relaxed breathing, begin loosening up the muscles of the feet by preliminary massage.

1. Wipe feet with cotton wool and an aromatherapy anti-septic toning lotion.
2. Holding foot firmly, rotate ankle clockwise then anti-clockwise slowly twice each way.
3. Rotate big toe twice each way.
4. With thumbs overlapped, zig-zag down sole of foot from toes to heel, then press firmly all the way up, keeping thumbs sideways.
5. With thumbs on sole of foot, and fingers on top, gently twist foot to the left, then to the right to spread tarsals.
6. Using whole hand, massage round ankle bone.
7. Using palm of hand, stroke firmly down inner side of sole.
8. Repeat 1-6 on other foot.
9. Gently rotate both thumbs over solar plexus reflexes, working on both feet at once, and without much pressure.
10. As in 2.

By this time the person should be well relaxed and ready for the reflex treatment.

Thumb Techniques
It is absolutely essential that thumb nails be very short indeed, especially on the outer edge, as one of the movements is done with the side of the thumb, the other being carried out with the ball of the thumb, so the top of the nail should also be filed back to 2 mm below the thumb pad. A combination of the two movements gives best benefits, and if the reflex is not easily reached by one method then the other can be tried. Whichever part of the thumb is being used the pressure is of the utmost importance – too little being unable to give a reaction on a tender reflex, yet too much being suddenly too painful on a tender one.

The foot itself should be held firmly by one hand and kept, without too much pressure, as forward as possible while the other thumb (with fingers resting on top of foot without using pressure) begins its search for reflexes.

Ball of Thumb.   With this method, pressure without any other movement is used on each point, the thumb is laid flat on the reflex area, and as pressure begins the thumb bends until at right angles. Relax so that thumb is ½ cm further on and repeat this caterpillar-like movement over the area.

Side of Thumb.   Here, the side of the thumb is placed on the reflex area and, while applying pressure, is rotated slightly, *without* moving over the skin. It is an on-the-spot movement with the side of the thumb then moved very slightly and the movement repeated. Sometimes it is easier to detect the crystals when the thumb is made to glide over a small area with pressure. A good example of this is from the bladder to the kidney, gliding up the ureter with pressure.

It is best to work through the body systems, completing wherever possible one system on both feet before beginning on the next. This not only keeps up the continuity of related reflexes but also is better than breaking off in the middle of the digestive system, say at the stomach, and starting again a few minutes after treating another reflex, e.g. kidney, on the way down the foot. This helps maintain equilibrium and relaxation induced in the body. (There are, of course, exceptions to every rule, and as an example it is easier to find the adrenal gland reflex when one has found the kidney reflex while doing the excretory system.)

When the person having treatment is sitting comfortably (or lying on a bed) put his other foot on a pillow on your knee and check that you, too, are in a comfortable position at a suitable height to reach his feet easily.

Remember that as you are looking at the feet in front of you the right foot is on your *LEFT* and the left foot is on your *RIGHT*. (See *Figure 9*.)

Carry out the foot relaxation technique on page 53 and check that the breathing is relaxed and even. Then follow the suggested routine below, as a diagnostic procedure only, noting which reflexes have a painful reaction. Even if the patient has told you his problem, still carry out a full diagnosis to check related organs. Each system must be found on *both* feet before going on to the next. (The exception is the digestive system where the instructions as specified in the order of work apply.)

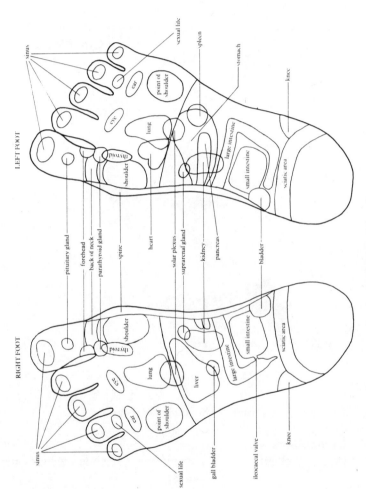

Figure 9. Reflexology chart.

Order of Work

1. **Nervous system:**

   Solar plexus — just under ball of foot, in centre (See *Figure 10.*)

   Sciatic nerve — (See *Figure 9.*)

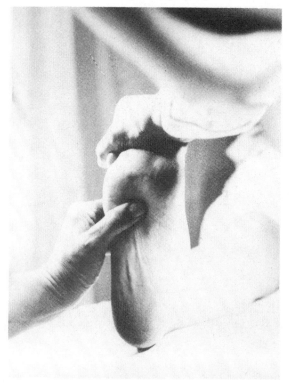

Figure 10. Solar plexus reflex

2. **Glandular system:**

   Pituitary gland — lower part of big toe cushion, in centre

   Parathyroid } — these two are very close to one
   Thyroid } another; thyroid usually treated as an area

   Sex gland — just under cushion of 4th toe

   Adrenal gland — top inside edge of kidney — best to do this reflex when doing kidney (See *Figure 14.*)

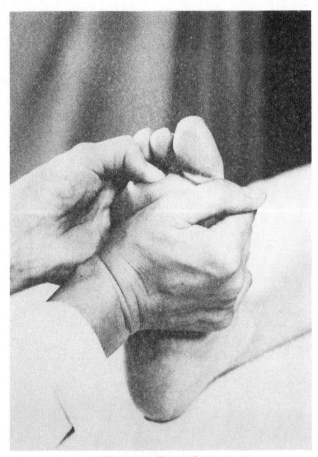

Figure 11. Eye reflex

3. Sinuses, Eye and Ear:

Sinuses   —   centre of cushion in each toe

Eye   —   between 2nd and 3rd toe *above* ball of foot, just *below* neck of toe (See *Figure 11*.)

Ear   —   same as above, but between toes 4 and 5

4. Bone and muscular system:

Spine   —   from big toe (cervical) to heel (coccyx) on inner edge of foot. Curve of foot relates to curve regions of spine. (See *Figure 12*.)

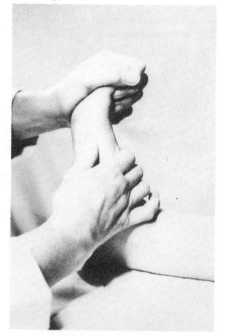

Figure 12. Part of spine reflex.

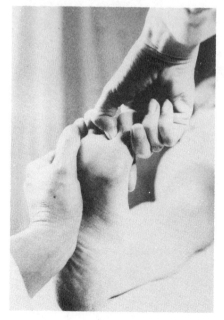

Figure 13. Neck reflex.

Neck	—	all round big toe neck (See *Figure 13*.)
Shoulder	—	main shoulder blade area found in fleshy part under big toe. Extremity of shoulder found just below neck of little toe.
Hip and knee	—	follow diagram (approximately on same level as bladder reflex but on little toe side of foot)

5. **Respiratory system:**

Lungs	—	large area on centre of ball of foot (diagram)

6. **Excretory system:**

Kidney	—	below solar plexus and slightly toward inside of foot. Kidney is

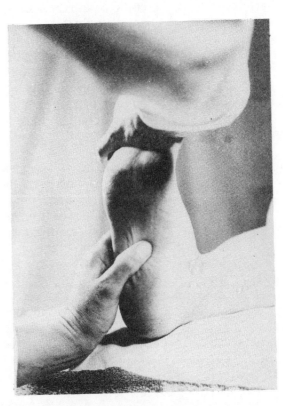

Figure 14. Kidney reflex.

easier to find if bladder is found first, then slide thumb up and slightly inwards on ureter tube until kidney reflex is felt. (See *Figure 14*.)

(Adrenal gland on top inside edge of kidney.)

Ureter — narrow area between kidney and bladder

Bladder — located on inside of foot near heel. Very often a little raised area on foot marks the spot.

7. **Digestive system:**

— stomach is mostly on left foot, also pancreas, but stomach entrance and the start of pancreas are on right foot, and this small area can be pressed if necessary after the liver and gall-bladder

Liver — large area on outside of foot, on your left hand side

Gall-bladder — on right hand lower edge of liver. Move to foot on right hand side.

Pancreas — along bottom edge of stomach reflex

Stomach — difficult, as so many organs overlap in this area. No problem to *treat*, but difficult to pinpoint which reflex is giving a reaction (see diagram). Try to keep to top right of stomach reflex.

Small intestine — below waist of foot — middle to inside edge; foot on your right first, then move to foot on your left.

Ileocaecal valve — still on your left, move towards large intestine.

Large intestine — carefully work upwards and along to waist of foot. Remember that as you pass kidney a reaction from *that* reflex may be felt. Continue across on to other foot, and complete.

8. Reproductive system:

Ovaries — between ankle bone and heel edge on little toe side of foot.

Fallopian Tube — approximately 1cm further up foot than groin gland, in a line between ankle bones.

Uterus — between ankle bone and heel edge on big toe side of foot. Work a little to each side also.

9. Circulatory system:

— this is helped with every reflex point pressed, but the heart can be gently massaged at the end of a treatment to make sure there is no blockage in the arteries, veins or valves in the heart, and to increase circulation.

Heart — found on left foot (right facing you) above and slightly to the left of the solar plexus.

Spleen — top right hand edge of stomach reflex.

Lymphatic system — follow diagram and cover all lymphatic points on each foot.
Note: The spleen and lymphatic system are included here because of their close relationship to the blood.

Having completed the diagnosis, return to the reflexes which showed a problem in that area, and treat as follows:

Treatment of Troubled Reflexes

It is usually more helpful to massage *all* the reflexes of the system in which the troubled reflex occurs, though obviously

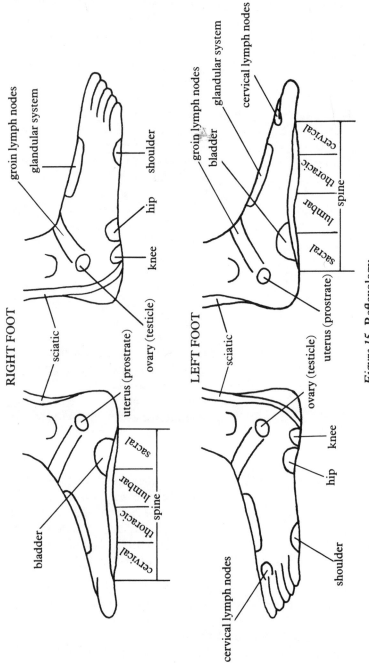

RIGHT FOOT

LEFT FOOT

groin lymph nodes
glandular system
shoulder
hip
knee
sciatic
uterus (prostrate)
ovary (testicle)
bladder
cervical
thoracic
lumbar
sacral
spine

groin lymph nodes
glandular system
cervical lymph nodes
bladder
sciatic
uterus (prostrate)
ovary (testicle)
cervical
thoracic
lumbar
sacral
spine
knee
hip
shoulder
cervical lymph nodes

Figure 15. Reflexology.

more time should be spent on the actual problem area. Other related areas can also be treated at the same time, e.g., the glandular system if that is felt to be the root cause of the other problem or problems.

Treatment involves a different concentration of pressure from diagnostic pressure, though the method of pressing is exactly the same. In diagnosis, pressure is used only to discover whether or not a blockage is present. Treatment is designed to break down and evenutally eliminate the blockage, so pressure is continued for a longer time on one place.

When treating a reflex, if the reaction is severe, the pressure should be relaxed sufficiently so that the person is not crying out with the pain (i.e., do not *over*treat) but do not relax enough so that no pain is felt at all. Some discomfort *should* be felt, otherwise no true treatment is being carried out. The pressure applied gradually breaks down the blockage in the energy pathway and it will be found that during half to one minute's massage the pain gradually diminishes, and it is necessary then to increase the pressure slightly until some discomfort is felt again. After another minute at that pressure it may be necessary to increase the pressure yet again. Never treat any one reflex for longer than three or four minutes.

You will know by the person's reactions the next day whether or not you have over or under treated. Over treatment, i.e. too heavy a pressure or too long a treatment, often makes someone feel worse the following day, but usually the day after that they feel much better. Under treatment, i.e. insufficient pressure to too short a treatment, simply results in no improvement at all. The correct pressure results in a definite improvement, however small, being felt.

After treatment is finished, for absolute optimum benefit essential oils should be chosen for the disorder shown, and mixed in 50 ml of carrier oil. (Refer to recipes section). This massage oil should be used to give a final relaxing massage to the feet, using effleurage* all over feet and legs up to the knee,plus movements 2, 6 and 7 from the preliminary massage, finishing with effleurage again.

The rest of the massage oil should be given to the person treated to rub into his feet, ankles and lower legs every night between treatments. The use of this massage oil (containing properly chosen essential oils) on a regular basis is not only

* See Chapter on Massage Techniques.

beneficial for any known disorder, but also plays an important preventative role, especially when movements 4 and 7 of the foot massage are included.

Reflexology done once a month on all reflexes, followed by the lower leg massage given below and using general tension essential oils (related if possible to any other disorder you may have found) is an excellent method of maintaining good health.

Lower leg massage:
1.   Apply a small amount of oil all over one leg (with the other leg wrapped in a towel to keep it warm).
2.   Effleurage up the front of the leg, using both hands with fingers facing one another and gently return down sides. Repeat 3 times.
3.   Effleurage up the back of the leg and return down sides 3 times.
4.   Effleurage firmly up back of leg, taking calf muscle to the side and returning to ankle. Repeat 4 times.
5.   Repeat, using other hand and taking muscle to the other side.
6.   Repeat, using each hand alternately and working a little further down the leg with each stroke, finishing on Achilles tendon.
7.   Do numbers 4, 6 and 7 from the foot massage.
8.   Repeat number 2.

6.

Simple Aromatherapy
Treatment Techniques

Before I explain the various treatment techniques possible with aromatherapy, I should like to point out a very important fact. We are all aware that any *one* form of treatment is not always totally effective on any one person, for any one particular problem, when used completely on its own.

For *some* people in certain circumstances and for *some* problems — yes — one form of treatment can succeed. But we must remember that it is not always as straightforward as that. Some people respond better to aromatherapy when combined with reflexology; others when they complement the massage treatment with home use of the essential oils in the bath or in their cups of tea. Some will benefit completely using only oils in the bath — others will not.

So we must have a sensible approach to the use of this important and interesting therapy and combine it with the other therapies mentioned in this book as and where necessary.

The easiest ways of using essential oils to help any disorder are:

1. taking them internally.
2. inhaling them.
3. putting them in the bath.
4. using them in a compress.

Internally. Daily ingestion of essential oil guarantees proper balance and functioning of intestines, and fights internal infections. They play a major role in the prevention of many diseases, including cancer. All aromatherapy doctors prescribe essential oils to be taken internally, either put into a glass of wine (red wine is the best) or to be taken with honey and water. My friend's mother, who lives in Aix-le-Provence in France, is treated *only* by an aromatherapy doctor and wouldn't go back to drugs and tablets. The only thing is, she says, it tastes like medicine, because essential oils are so concentrated!

If a short dose is preferred, then the glass of wine or honey and water method is best. For the latter take 1 teaspoonful of honey and add 1 to 2 teaspoonsful of boiling water to dissolve it. To either the wine or the honey mixture add 1 to 3 drops of the chosen essential oil or oils, and swallow. If you are very brave, just drop the essential oil on to a sugar lump and eat it! You should have 2 to 3 doses per day, depending on your problem.

Another way of taking oils internally is by making a 'tea', using tea bags and essential oil. This too, should be taken 2 to 3 times per day. Experiment with different 'flavours', choosing carefully from the oils you need.

Make a pot of tea using one tea bag only, and after 2 minutes stir and remove the tea bag. Add 2 drops of essential oil and pour a cupful. I prefer these teas without milk or sugar, but try with sugar if preferred. If milk *has* to be used, the tea must be made with 2 tea bags and then follow instructions as for one bag.

Any essential oil can be used, following the therapeutic index on page 103, and two or three can be mixed together in a small dropper bottle to be used as required, when you find a mixture you like.

By the way, Earl Grey tea is just ordinary tea with essential oil of bergamot in it, and I often put 2 drops of bergamot into my teapot if I have no Earl Grey tea!

The following is only a selection of the ailments which can be treated internally:

coughs and colds	headaches and painful periods
flatulence	cystitis
indigestion	depression
constipation	varicose veins
diarrhoea	stones in the kidney or urinal tract.

Inhalations. These are recommended for those people who cannot take medicines or don't enjoy essential oil tea.

One of the easiest ways to inhale essential oils is simply to put about 10 drops on a paper towel or handkerchief and keep inhaling from it. Put one on your pillow, beside your nose, at nights — with nasal congestion it is an ideal way to ensure a free breathing passage during the night.

Another way of inhaling is to put essential oils into hot water and breathe the vapour which comes from it. This time the 10 drops of essential oil should be put in 100 ml of hot water. It is best to put a towel over your head and the basin, to keep the vapour in a small area. Breathe in deeply (preferably through the nose) until the smell has almost disappeared. This treatment should be repeated 3 times a day.

Madame Maury used to use inhalations for her clients, between aromatherapy body massage treatments, and found it successful for many of the complaints brought to her salon.

Inhalations are mainly used for:

tension   headaches

disorders relating to the respiratory tract, e.g.,
colds   sore throat
blocked sinuses   cough, etc.

Foot and Hand Baths. This treatment is a nice easy one to do while sitting down at night. All that is needed is a bowl of hand-hot water with 8 to 10 drops of essential oil. Keep a kettle of just-boiled water beside the bowl to add to the water if it goes too cool. Steep hands or feet for 10 to 15 minutes, moving them around every now and again. Wrap in a dry towel after soaking, and leave for another 15 minutes. Finish the treatment by massaging into your feet and lower legs a little massage oil containing some essential oils. (See page 64)

Troubles which benefit best with a bath treatment are:

rheumatism   dermatitis
arthritis   dry skin, etc.

Baths. The bath should be hand-hot before adding the essential oils and 10 drops in ½ bath of water, 15 in ¾ bath of water, are the amounts needed. One should stay in the bath for at least 15 minutes, turning over if possible half way through. (Not necessary when water completely covers body). Essential oil baths are very pleasant to have, and most beneficial.

Conditions benefiting from baths:

insomnia   menstruation problems
nervous tension   coughs and colds
muscular disorders   headaches
circulation problems   fluid retention, etc.

Compresses. Very useful as a treatment for skin problems, bruises, muscular and chest pains, and indeed can be used over a problem area for disorders such as painful periods.

The normal strength for compresses is 10 drops in 100 ml as for inhalations, but I have used 2 or 3 drops neat on a gauze for a bad bruise with excellent results.

Old sheeting in four thicknesses is ideal for a compress, cut large enough to cover the area being treated. Do not use *medicated* lint or gauze, but untreated cotton wool in the roll can be used for small areas. However, remember that cotton wool is more absorbent than sheeting and will probably soak up more liquid, so do bear this, and the size of the compress, in mind when mixing the essential oils. For example 200 ml with 10 drops may be needed for a large area, but a small area may only take 50 ml of water, but still 10 drops of essential oil. It is the concentration of oil onto or into the body that counts therapeutically, as will be seen later when oils are mixed for massage.

Pour enough measured hot water into a bowl to be soaked up in the size of compress chosen for the treatment. (Experiment and practice will soon make it easy to determine the quantity necessary) and add 10 drops of essential oils (chosen from the therapeutic cross reference on page 132.)

Put the compress into the water and essential oils, and squeeze out so that it will not drip, but not enough to make it nearly dry.

Place the compress over the area being treated, and wrap a sheet of thin plastic around it. To help the compress to work more efficiently put a pre-warmed towel and blanket over the top to keep the compress warm. Ideally, leave on for two hours (at least). For the back, apply the compress in reverse order; warm towel on bed, then plastic sheet, then compress; and then lie on it and cover the top of the body with a warm blanket.

Occasionally, and for a tiny area, a compress using neat essential oils is very beneficial, for example, sprains, bruises, wounds, neuralgia, abscesses, etc. Here, the neat oil is put onto the area and can be covered with damp gauze or cotton wool, which can then be kept on the skin by the use of micropore surgical tape.

Conditions benefiting best from compresses are:

skin problems	painful periods
neuralgia	sprains
bruises	muscular aches and pains
open wounds	

Neat essential oils are also very beneficial in an emergency such as a burn, nettle rash, scald or insect bite to ease the initial discomfort and act as an antiseptic. In these cases they do not need to be covered; just apply neat essential oil at regular intervals and leave. Herpes, though not an emergency, responds wonderfully to neat application of essential oil.

Massage. This is a most useful form of aromatherapy, and gives great benefit to almost any condition. Being so important, the next two chapters are devoted to this subject.

7.

An Explanation of Massage

The field of massage has widened considerably over the last ten to twenty years, incorporating new types of massage such as shiatsu and reflexology, although these last two are mainly concerned with *pressure* rather than *massage* as we understand it.

In body massage pressure is, of course, used, but in many different ways. The nearest movement in a western massage to shiatsu and reflexology pressure is the first part only of what we call thumb frictions, where pressure is put on certain parts of the body, with the thumbs, before making small circles over that area.

The word 'massage' comes from a Greek word meaning to *knead*, and it is one of the oldest forms of treatment for human ailments. Hippocrates (460-380 BC) said about a dislocated shoulder — 'it is necessary to rub the shoulder gently and smoothly with soft hands. The physician must be experienced in many things, but assuredly also in rubbing.' Various systems and techniques have been developed over the years and people with many and varied qualifications have prescribed and performed massage.

The effects of massage treatment naturally depend greatly upon the technical skill and knowledge of the masseur or masseuse. Through proper and skilful massage all the functions of the organs of the body — skin, muscles, nerves, glands, etc. are stimulated, and by the increased circulation of the blood and lymph, the clearing away of body waste is assisted.

Body massage movements can vary from soft, light, rhythmical stroking movements designed to relax the muscles and nerves, to heavy pounding and kneading designed to break up fatty areas.

In aromatherapy we use mostly stroking movements, or effleurage as it is called, a little kneading and some frictions (called compression), and it is as well to understand these before trying to help anyone.

Effleurage

(a) Superficial stroking: used always in the return direction from deep stroking, but can be used on its own. Over large areas the palms (and fingers) of the hand are used and they should relax to the shape of the body underneath them, in other words, mould themselves to the part of the body being massaged.

(b) Deep stroking: this is done with the whole hand as in superficial stroking, but it is done with pressure and always in the direction of the heart. (This helps the venous flow). It is only done in that direction, the return journey always being a light, superficial stroke.

When doing effleurage, the hands should keep in contact with the body all the time, and the rhythm of the strokes should be slow and even.

Effleurage improves venous flow, i.e., helps to remove congestion in the veins. Because of this the fresh blood can circulate more freely, taking nutrients to all the organs through which it passes. The absorption of waste products is hastened and the lymphatic circulation improved. As an added bonus, it is extremely soothing and relaxing, particularly for nervous, irritated or over-tired people.

Compression

(a) Petrissage (or kneading). This is when a muscle, part of a muscle or a muscle group is picked up and squeezed or rolled, then released while the other hand moves to the adjacent area to repeat the process. This movement is usually done with both hands, using the palm and whole length of the fingers, or the thumb and fingers, depending on the size of the muscle area being massaged. It is essential that this movement is carried out only after the area has been previously relaxed by effleurage, and it should be slow, gentle and rhythmical, always returning to starting point without a break in contact or with a superficial stroke.

Petrissage increases the circulation and the removal of waste products, thus helping fatigue. The skin, deep and superficial or 'surface' tissues are all stimulated into further activity. The sudden releasing of the stretched muscle fibres causes them to contract momentarily, thus strengthening them, and finally, fat and fibrous tissues can sometimes be broken down.

(b) Frictions (or deep rubbing in circles). These movements can be carried out with the palm of the hand, the cushions of the thumbs or one or more fingers. With frictions, it is as though the part of the hand being used is 'stuck' to the skin on the body being massaged: the skin must move, *with* the part of the hand being used, *over* the tissues beneath, with pressure. After several circles over one area have been completed, the pressure is released so that the hand (*without losing contact*) can glide to the next area and the movement be repeated. Pressure must be firm but not so heavy that it may cause injury to the underlying tissues.

Frictions aid the removal of excess fluid in the body and stimulate the circulation. Most importantly, they can some-times break down fat, fibrous thickenings and tension nodules in the part being treated.

There is another form of body massage used called **Percussion** which, as the name suggests, is made up of short, sharp movements. There are many types of percussion (with names like pounding, hacking, cupping, etc!) but none of them are used in aromatherapy, as none are relaxing.

You can see how important it is for massage movements to be done correctly, and how the best results are obviously obtained by visiting a qualified masseur. However, as in all arts, such as cooking, painting, pottery etc., certain people without profes-sional training possess a natural ability to carry out these arts, and with just a little help, to make sure the technique is correct, these people can attain quite a good standard. It is for *this type of person* that I have given such detailed descriptions of the massage movements. They will, with the assistance of essential oils, be able to help their relatives and friends in a completely natural and harmless way, with no risk of side effects.

Reminders

Do not massage if an infection of any sort is present, or if there is a fracture in the area.

Massage *gently* and carefully over recent scar tissue and varicose veins, both of which can be helped by choosing the right essential oils and using only effleurage, to aid the penetration of the oils. (Both conditions can be harmed by heavy and incorrect massage techniques).

During pregnancy massage is recommended on any part of the body up to the fourth or fifth month. After this time it would not be comfortable to lie face downwards, so only massage areas which do not involve this position.

Do not massage heavily over bruised or broken skin, but do treat these with essential oils either by a compress or very lightly massaging neat oils into the affected area.

8.

Aromatherapy Massage Techniques

Always make sure that the room you are working in is warm, and that your nails are short. Many small area massage treatments, like shoulders, can be done in the living room, but if you are wanting to cover the whole back, or legs, then a firm bed in a warm bedroom is essential. Better still, use a table with blankets, or a strip of foam for comfort.

I will start with the back massage; it is the longest and most complicated, but it is easier to practice the movements on a larger area, and having become familiar with the basic movements, you will find it easier to adapt for special smaller tension areas. Miss out all numbers with * beside them to start with, and add these as you become more proficient and confident.

It is important that the person being massaged is breathing out whenever shiatsu pressures are being done, also massage on the abdomen, which involves pressure. The breathing should just be adjusted, and quite normal, not exaggerated.

Choose the essential oils needed and mix them in a 50 ml bottle of blended carrier oils, (grapeseed oil and wheatgerm or avocado if needed) as explained in Chapter 9.

Back Massage

1. Put about a teaspoonful of massage oil in the palm of one hand. Rub both hands together lightly, then spread the oil over the whole back with wide sweeping effleurage movements.
2. Put hands at base of spine, fingers facing shoulders all the time; and stroke firmly up each side of spine, using the whole hand, round the shoulder blade, then very lightly down the back to the base of spine. Repeat 4 or 5 times. (See *Figure 16*.)
3. Put one hand over the other (reinforced hand) to give strength to the next movement — still at base of spine. Push firmly up one side of back to shoulder area, where hands cross the spine upwards between the shoulder

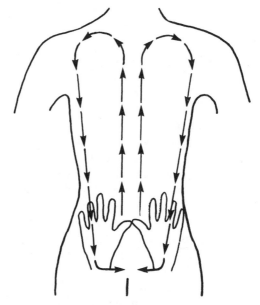

Figure 16. Movement 2 (back).

blades, go right round the shoulder, cross the spine upwards and go right round the other shoulder, making a figure eight movement. Repeat the figure eight 4 or 5 times, bringing hands back to base of spine on the last repeat. During this movement keep the *whole* of the reinforced hand on the body. (See *Figures 17 and 18.*)

4*. Pressures down bladder meridians (breathing). Stroke firmly with hands up back to neck from finishing point in No. 3 and turn them to place both thumbs together and facing one another in the spinal channel at left side of spine (about 1 or 2 cm from spine itself). Press firmly down with thumbs and release. Move one thumb's width further down channel and repeat. Repeat right down to hip level. Slide gently back to top of channel, and keeping thumbs together slide with pressure (no special breathing) first the left, then right thumb about 2 cm at a time, i.e., slide left and bring right to meet it. Repeat down to hip level. Repeat whole movement on right side of spine. (See *Figures 19 and 20.*)

5. Place hands as for movement 2 and push firmly up back with whole hands, going right round shoulder blades but not returning to base of spine. Go round shoulder

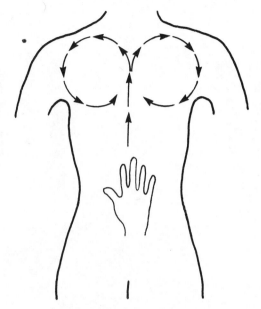

Figure 17. Movement 3 (back).

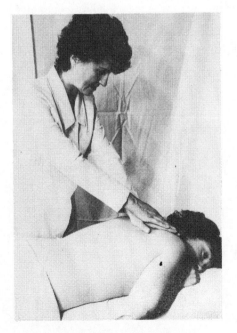

Figure 18. Movement 3 (back).

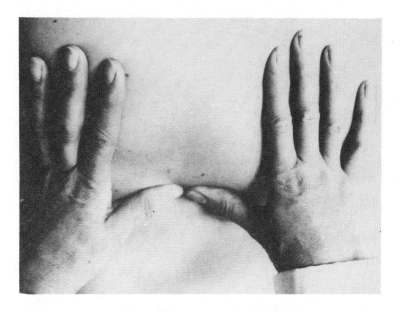

Figure 19. Movement 4 (back) showing position of thumbs in one spinal channel (one thumb facing head, one thumb facing feet).

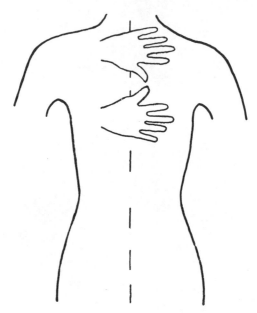

Figure 20. Movement 4 (back).

blades again, finishing the circle a little lower down the back. Repeat shoulder blade circle, finishing this time just above waist level. Repeat, finishing a little lower down each time until the last circle finishes at the base of the spine, having covered the whole of the back in one cirle. (See *Figure 21*.)

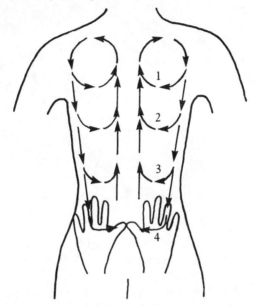

Figure 21. Movement 5 (back).

6. Hands as for movement 2 and push straight up back over tops of shoulders, returning very lightly and without pressure. Repeat twice.
7. Push up and back and out towards armpits, returning by same path but without pressure. Repeat twice.
8. Push up back and out to chest, returning lightly as before. Repeat twice.
9*. Do first half of No. 4 as far as thumbs facing one another on left side. Let thumbs overlap as finger lengths squeeze together and release once, quickly and lightly, moving their length towards armpit and repeating the squeeze, and release. Move and repeat twice. Now move one hand's width down back, and starting again near spine repeat squeeze and release four times towards side of body. Move hands and repeat once more at waist level. (See *Figure 22*.)

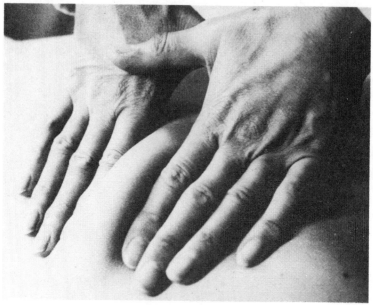

Figure 22. Movement 9 (back).

10. Slide back to top of spine and place finger pads in a *straight* line in left spinal channel. Press firmly and push fingers out to armpits with pressure. Move one hand's width down back and repeat. Repeat twice more. Now repeat whole movement on right side of back. (See *Figure 23.*)

11. Repeat No. 2 four times.

12★. Effleurage up left side of back, from hip level to shoulders. Use alternate hands, pushing with fingers facing shoulders at spine side, moving out towards side of body and opening fingers as you do so. The next hand comes underneath the first one and repeats the movement; each hand moves up the body a little as well as going sideways like a fan. Finish at shoulder with hand nearest head while the other comes in again at hip level to start again. Repeat three times. Repeat whole movement on right side. (See *Figure 24.*)

13. Using thumbs, do friction circles from waist on either side of spine, out and round hip bone. Repeat three times, each time doing a smaller curve. (See *Figures 25 and 26.*)

14. Repeat No. 2 four or five times.

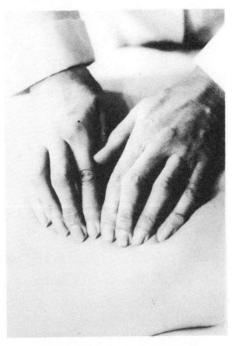

Figure 23. Movement 10 (back).

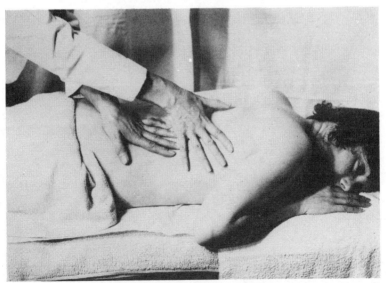

Figure 24. Movement 12 (back).

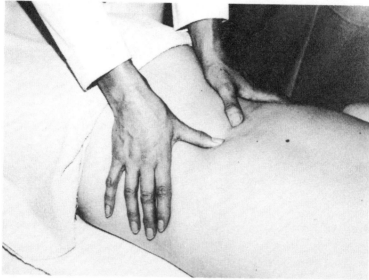

Figure 25. Movement 13 (back).

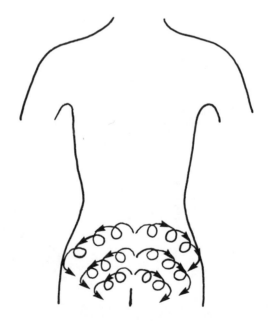

Figure 26. Movement 13 (back).

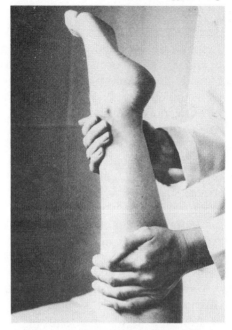

Figure 27. Movement 3 (back of leg).

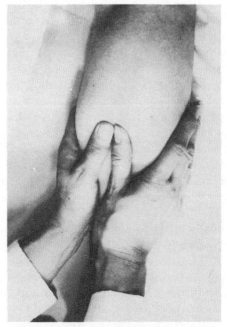

Figure 28. Movement 4 (back of leg).

Back of Legs

1. Put a small amount (about ½ teaspoonful) of mixed oil into the palm of one hand. Rub both hands together lightly, and spread oil over the whole of back leg.
2. Stand at side of bed and place hands across one ankle (fingers facing out to side of body and palms on top of leg). Let fingers fall gently to shape of leg at the side. Effleurage firmly towards thigh, taking hand nearest to top of leg all the way up to top of thigh; then hand nearest feet to back of knee. Continue this alternate stroking one way only, and without losing contact with leg between strokes, five or six times.
3. Lift foot up with one hand and with the other stroke with pressure from ankle to knee on back of leg, keeping palm in centre and fingers relaxed round leg. Repeat four of five times. (See *Figure 27*.)
4. Stand at bottom of bed and slide thumbs up leg from ankle to knee firmly, with pressure, and return with light effleurage down sides of leg. (See *Figure 28*.)
5. Repeat movement 2 five or six times.
6. Repeat all movements on other leg.

Front of Legs

1. Put oil on as before.
2. With hands facing opposite ways but close together, effleurage firmly up whole of leg and lightly return down sides, sandwiching foot as shown.
   Repeat three or four times, finishing with an extra half movement to top of thigh. (See *Figures 29 and 30*.)
3. Turn body so that hands face towards ankle. Stroke lightly down sides of thigh to knee. There, apply pressure and lift up towards middle of top leg, stroking firmly to top of thigh with whole hand. Repeat three times. (See *Figure 31*.)
4. Stroke firmly from inside leg at knee to outside, diagonally upwards and using alternate hands until top of leg is reached. Return to knee without a break, and repeat three or four times.
5. Bring hands down to knee, but facing upwards, and make a bridge of your first fingers and thumbs. Push these over the knee cap and return down sides of knee area with whole of hands. Repeat four or five times, returning to the foot at least once.

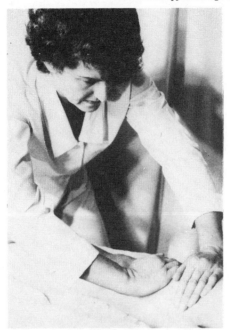

Figure 29. Movement 2a (front of leg).

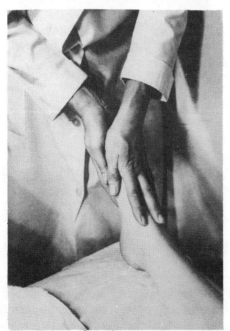

Figure 30. Movement 2b (front of leg).

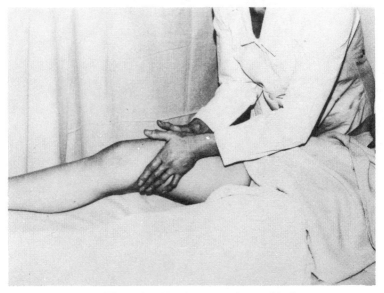

Figure 31. Movement 3 (front of leg).

6. Repeat movement 2 three or four times.

A simple massage of the lower leg is given in detail in the Reflexology chapter; this is useful when the whole leg does not need a massage.

Abdomen

Massage of the abdomen (or hara) is called ampuku therapy in the East, and is excellent for ensuring general well-being, relaxation and good digestion.

No pressures are ever done with the thumbs in ampuku therapy; pressure points are covered during massage carried out with the palm of the hand and fingers and whenever pressure *is* applied, using these, the recipient should be breathing out.

1. Apply a small amount of oil all over tummy and up to rib cage.
2. Place hands with overlapping fingers pointing towards head exactly where chest bone ends and outside edges lying against (but not on) rib cage. Pull hands down and out towards waist, turning fingers so that they go under the body; pause; lift firmly upwards and pull hands

down and inwards (outside edge lying against hip bones this time) to pelvic bone.

Repeat this diamond shaped movement 3 or 4 times. (See *Figure 32.*)

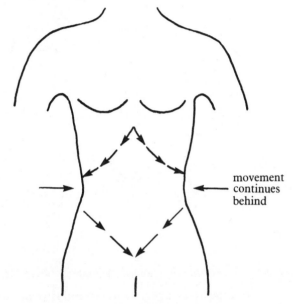

movement
continues
behind

Figure 32. Movement 2 (abdomen).

3. Using the outside edge of both hands alternately, stroke down left rib cage and then right rib cage.
4. With reinforced palms of hands do small circles in one big circle about 7½ cm from navel, slowly in a clockwise direction.
5. Find the Tan Den point; take the person's fingers, bend his or her elbow and place the index finger over the navel. Immediately where ring finger finishes, in line with the navel, is the Tan Den point, the seat of all general tension and the emotions. Place the length of your middle finger over this spot and reinforce it with the middle finger of the other hand. Without poking, massage in gentle clockwise circles on this spot, not moving over the skin, but stuck to the skin and moving *it* over the underlying tissue. If you find this difficult, or uncomfortable for the person receiving the massage, use the palm of your hand, reinforced with the other one, over the general area. (See *Figure 33.*)

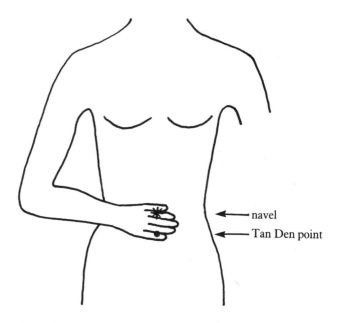

Figure 33. Movement 5 (abdomen) to find the Tan Den point.

6. Effleurage up centre tummy, round rib cage and return down sides of body.
7. Repeat No. 2.

Scalp

This is very relaxing for anyone who suffers from headaches and is best done with oil on your fingers from doing another part of the body. Oil put on the hands specially is often lost on the hair itself.

1. Stand above person's head and place fingers all round hairline as far as you can. Move up round hairline then through hair towards top of head to a comfortable position to draw your fingers out through hair. Repeat five or six times. (See *Figure 34*.)
2. Hold all fingers in contact with scalp, as though stuck with glue and move fingers *and* scalp over the bone beneath. (Do not move fingers through hair *over* scalp). Change position and repeat. Change and repeat until all scalp has had friction massage.
3. Repeat No. 1.

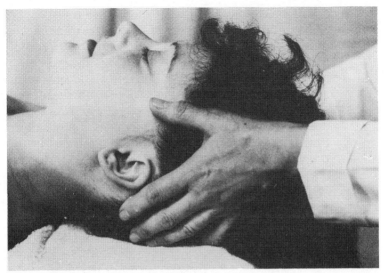

Figure 34. Movement 1 (scalp).

Face
The pressures in this massage are very good for headaches, eyestrain, sinuses and head colds. People with bronchitis or chest colds are helped tremendously by reflexology on the reflexes for sinuses, eyes and ears, spine, shoulders, neck and lungs, followed by aromatherapy massage using the right oils on the feet and legs, face and back. Numbers 3, 5 and 7 can be done on oneself for headaches, sinus or head colds to relieve congestion.

1. Put a very small amount of mixed oil into the palm of one hand. Rub both hands together and apply oil lightly all over the face, neck and upper chest.
2. Do gentle, upward effleurage on face and neck, with both hands. Include light circles round eyes (starting in direction of eyebrows), using ring fingers, and stroke up forehead with alternate hands (fingers lying across forehead), finishing by sliding both hands (turning fingers as you go, to face downwards) to temples, where gentle but firm pressure should be given.
3. Keeping fingers gently on sides of head, about ear level, place both thumbs one on top of the other on centre forehead between eyebrows. Press downwards firmly and move one thumb's width higher up. Repeat three or four times up to hairline.

4. Stroke up the same area with alternate thumbs.
5. Still keeping fingers on sides of head, place thumbs side by side between eyebrows. Press firmly and release. Move one thumb's width along top of eyebrows, towards temples, and repeat. Do this whole movement twice more. Move one thumb's width *up* forehead, and with thumbs together again in centre forehead repeat pressures, moving out towards temples. Repeat these rows once or twice more until the last one is just below the hairline. (See *Figure 35.*)

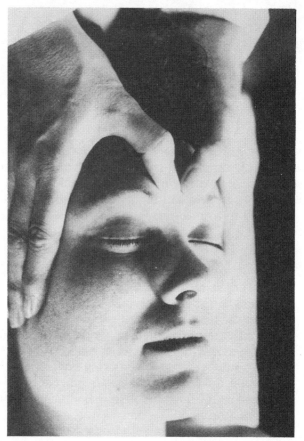

Figure 35. Movement 5 (face).

6. Still keeping fingers on sides of head place the big muscle of thumbs (thenar muscle) to meet in the centre forehead (thumbs pointing towards chin) press and

slide out to temples. Repeat three or four times. (See *Figure 36.*)

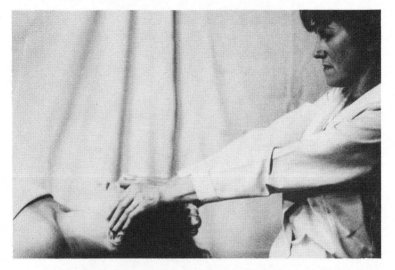

Figure 36. Movement 6 (face) and movement 9c (face).

7. Place thumbs on forehead and with second and third fingers press and release on top of cheekbone on sides of nose, move one finger's width outwards, and press and release again. Repeat the pressures, following the crescent shape of the cheek bone, until almost at temples. Move one finger's width *down* the face and repeat the pressures, still keeping the crescent shape. If there is room, repeat again. (See *Figure 37.*)

8. Return to top of nose, press and slide out to temples with pressure, keeping the crescent shape. Move down one finger's width, and repeat; and again.

9*. Place index fingers on top lip, middle and ring fingers below lips and, hugging the face with all the hand, pull out and up towards temple. Leave fingers on temple, lean back and place thumb muscles onto centre forehead, and slide with pressure to meet the fingers, still at the temples. Lift up the fingers and leaving the thenar muscle on the temples lean forward and repeat the whole movement three or four times more. (See *Figures 38, 39 and 40.*)

10. Follow *Figure 41.* for the shiatsu pressure points — in each case use ring or middle fingers. The fingers should

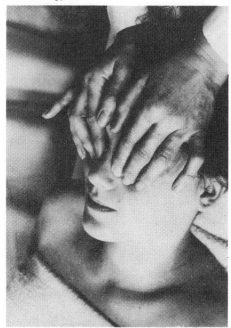

Figure 37. Movement 7 (face).

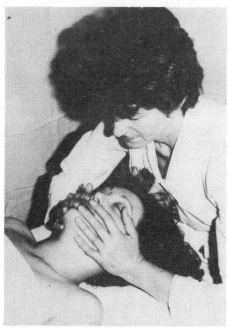

Figure 38. Movement 9a (face).

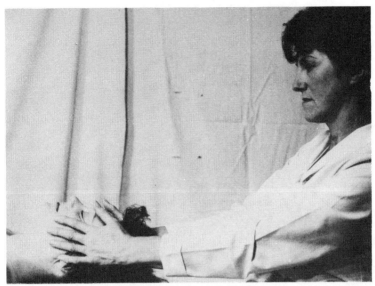

Figure 39. Movement 9b (face).

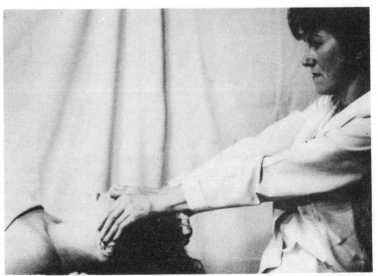

Figure 40. Movement 6 (face) and Movement 9c (face).

(and will with experience) find a little hollow to slip into, and then pressure at right angles to pressure point is applied and slowly released.

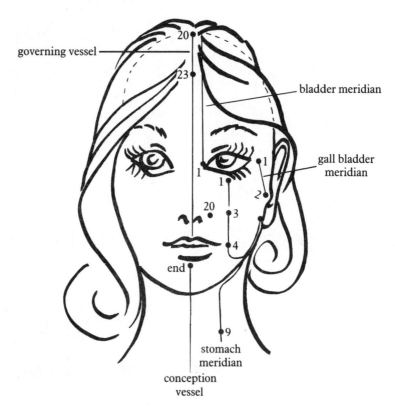

Figure 41. Pressure points of the face.

All points need not be covered, e.g., one could just do the following selection from the facial section of the Pressure Point Identification Table on page 41.

> just behind mouth corners
> about 2½ cm in front of ear lobe base, just below jaw bone
> between lower lip and chin (press with one finger on top of the other)
> just above inside corner of eye, on bone; press upwards
> about 2½ cm from outside corner of eye right on temples; feel until a little hollow is found.

11. Repeat No. 2, including this time effleurage from top of neck down to and across chest, round shoulder blades and back to top of neck. Finish with eye and forehead stroking, this time making the alternate forehead strokes slower and slower, until you no longer put the second hand onto the head, but just bring the other very slowly off, the little finger being the last thing to leave the forehead.

Arms
These can best be done in a sitting position.
1. Spread the oil over the arms in the usual way, and (holding the hand with one hand) do effleurage strokes over the whole arm with the other. Change hands and do the inside arm.
2. Friction movements can be done where there are problem areas, e.g., rheumatism or arthritis, adapting whatever is suitable from movements already learnt.
3. Stroke up centre palm with thumbs (supporting hand with fingers behind) over the thenar* muscle and outer side of hand.
4. Do zig-zag movements down palm with whole of thumbs and push firmly back up towards wrist.
5. Do zig-zags on both sides of wrist.
6. Effleurage on back of hand with whole of thumbs.
7. Repeat effleurage in No. 1.

Shoulders
Quite often there is tension in the upper neck and shoulder area, extending to base of shoulder blade. This is sometimes easier to treat in a sitting position where you can get right on top of the shoulder itself and do kneading or petrissage there.
1. Apply oil in the usual way and do soothing effleurage strokes around shoulder blades.
2. Using thumbs do alternate strokes just to left hand side of spine up to neck and up neck itself to hairline if necessary.
3. Pick up, squeeze and release top shoulder muscle from shoulder edge along to neck.

* Big thumb muscle on side of palm.

4. Do alternate strokes with thumbs up top of shoulder towards neck and up neck if necessary.
5. Using thumbs again do friction massage over any nodules in the shoulders themselves.
6. Repeat the effleurage in No. 1.

9.

Preparing Oils for Massage

We have to have some medium with which to carry out massage movements — something to help our hands to move over the skin evenly. Some masseurs use talcum powder, but this can be very drying; most use some form of vegetable or mineral oil. For the massage movements alone to be effective, any of the three mediums can be used. But for aromatherapy it is necessary to choose something which will 'carry' the chosen essential oils (which themselves are not, despite their name, oily or greasy) through the skin and into the blood circulation. . . so we have to use oil rather than powder.

Mineral oil is useless, because although essential oils will dissolve in it, it has a very low penetration power (hence its use as baby oil) so the essential oil is restricted in its attempt to pass through the skin.

Certain fine vegetable oils are ideal, as they are of themselves fairly penetrative and therefore do not hinder the highly penetrative

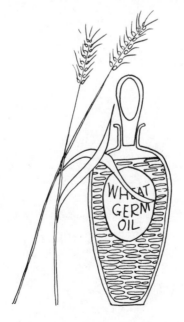

essential oils from getting into the blood stream. It is essential that a pure, good quality and very fine oil is chosen as a carrier to hasten the curative effects of the essential oils you put into it. Only just enough is needed to be able to move smoothly over the area being massaged. If too much is used, you will slip or slide over the area, wasting the oil and not doing much good with your movements.

There are several good vegetable oil bases which can be used for blending. The choice is dependent partly on the smell (it should have little or no smell), partly on the texture of the oil, and partly on price.

All carrier oils used must of course be 100 per cent pure for maximum penetration, and usually the higher the price the more pure it is, and the better the keeping quality.

Avocado and hazelnut oils possibly penetrate the skin the most easily; avocado and wheatgerm oils are the most nourishing; grapeseed, olive, peachnut, sweet almond, sweetcorn, soya bean and sunflower seed oils are all good basic oils, not varying a great deal in effect, but varying in aroma (very important — there should be none), penetration, price (quite a lot), and keeping qualities (also very important).

As a basic carrier oil I prefer grapeseed oil. It is very clear, exceptionally fine and without any smell — in other words it fulfils all the requirements of a good basic oil. Added to that, it happens to

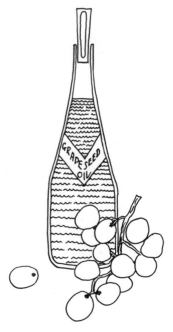

be one of the least expensive, so that is an added bonus.

Grapeseed (or any of the basic oils) can be used on its own, but if a bottle of massage oil is being made up for daily use, then 5 per cent of wheatgerm oil (which is an anti-oxidant), should be added to help the keeping qualities; sweetcorn oil is not a good choice, as its keeping qualities are the least good. Vegetable oils on their own keep fairly well, but once essential oils have been added they tend to oxidize and turn rancid, so never mix more than a couple of months supply (50-100 ml) at any one time, and always add 5 per cent of wheatgerm oil to the mix.

Wheatgerm oil is also good for a dry skin, and the percentage used can be increased if wished, but it is rarely used on its own as it is too rich, too heavy and also more expensive!

Avocado is another rich, heavier and more expensive carrier oil which is rarely used on its own. It, too, is good for a dry skin, but it is added to grapeseed usually to help penetration, as its penetrative powers (along with hazelnut oil) are greater than other carrier oils. So 5 per cent can be added to the mix for speedier penetration or if the person being massaged has a lot of fatty tissue.

So it is possible for a 50ml bottle of carrier oil to be made up as follows:

1 teaspoonful wheatgerm oil
1 teaspoonful avocado or hazelnut oil $\left.\right\}$ into bottle
Fill up with grapeseed (or other basic carrier oil).
It is then ready to add the therapeutic element:
the essential oils.

Adding Essential Oils

It is important to select the correct quantity of essential oil to put into the carrier oil. This depends to a large extent on the area to be covered during any one treatment. True aromatherapy, as carried out by beauty therapists and physiotherapists, is a *total* treatment, and should be carried out on the face, scalp, body, legs and arms. When you are helping a particular ailment yourself you can do the part of the body giving the problem.

What you have to remember then is that the amount of blended oil used is going to go right round the body, carried by the blood, and if the same concentration is used on a back alone as is used on a whole body, there may not be enough essential oil in the bloodstream to give a sufficiently effective result. So you need to add between 15 and 30 drops to a 50ml bottle of oil, because at any one time you will only be using about a teaspoonful of oil, therefore the essential oil percentage going into your bloodstream at each massage will be very small — the equivalent of 2 or 3 drops.

It is worth mentioning here that a few essential oils have normalizing effects; i.e., they will sedate or uplift, relax or stimulate, and will successfully treat an oily or a dry skin. The result obtained depends on the condition of the person being treated.

. A minute proportion of the chosen oils can effect a cure, as in the case of digitalis mentioned earlier. Usually, the more toxic the essence the smaller should be the quantity used. Sage and fennel are relatively more toxic than most oils. Rose, lavender and camomile have a very low toxicity. None on our list are very toxic.

Some problems respond better to a very dilute essential oil, where others, requiring the same oil to be used for the treatment, may need a greater strength to respond positively. It will be found that trial and error sometimes play a very big part in determining the concentration of oil to use for a particular person for a specific complaint.

This is confusing to the beginner but expertise and confidence will soon be acquired by experience. It is best initially to use the average percentage given or less, and only if this does not give the desired result should the concentration be increased. It does not necessarily follow that the more you use the better will be the effect — in fact *it is often the reverse*.

Lower concentrations often give as good or better results if the problem is emotional, but if you are working mainly on a physical problem then a higher concentration would probably produce better results.

10.

Recipes

The table on page 110 gives a description of many of the essential oils available, with a list of their uses. The most popular, useful and interesting oils have been included. The list is in three sections: top note oils, which are mainly stimulating and uplifting; middle note oils, which cover most bodily ailments; and base note oils, which are mainly sedative.

The most useful reference list, however, is the therapeutic index of selected problems on page 132 and it will be found invaluable for information concerning the oils to treat a specific condition.

Therapeutically, most of the problems one comes up against can be dealt with by the less expensive oils (lavender is particularly useful), and camomile, but jasmine, neroli (orange blossom) and rose are unbeatable for their delightful aromas and excellent effects on complaints of nervous origin, e.g., tension, anxiety and stress.

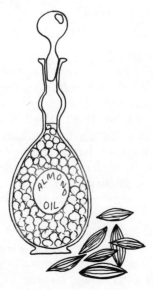

Essential oils can be used in several ways, to make a tea, to use in the bath, to mix in a massage oil, etc. If you want to use the essential oils in all these ways it is beneficial to use a 10ml dropper bottle and mix, say, 20 drops each of the oils you have chosen for your condition (let us assume muscle cramp) so that you have a ready mixed treatment bottle (which you must label 'cramp') of pure essential oils from which you make your tea, add to carrier oils for massage, put in the bath, etc.

And now we come to the exciting part! Selecting which oils to use!

You will find when you turn to the therapeutic index not only that several oils will treat one symptom, but also that one oil will treat several symptoms, so first of all write down the condition you are wanting to treat the most, e.g., you may be suffering from rheumatism, and migraine. Decide which condition gives you the most discomfort. Let us suppose it is the migraine. Now write down all the essential oils which treat migraine (see the Therapeutic Index).

'migraine: basil, eucalyptus, camomile, lavender, marjoram, melissa, peppermint, rosemary, rose'

Well, we can't use all of those! If you suffer from migraine alone, then choose from the above oils any one oil or up to four (never more than four) to get the right aroma for you. But as we want to treat your rheumatism as well if we can, turn to 'rheumatism' and see if any of the oils for migraine repeat themselves.

'rheumatism: eucalyptus, lemon, sage, thyme, camomile, juniper, hyssop, lavender, marjoram, rosemary'

So eucalyptus, camomile, lavender, marjoram and rosemary will treat both your rheumatism *and* your migraine. First of all, put one drop of any two or three oils into a teaspoonful of carrier oil (in an egg cup), mix and rub a little onto the back of your hand. Does it smell nice? If you like it, those are the oils to use. If you have used eucalyptus or camomile and they are too predominant, put in one extra drop of either lavender, marjoram or rosemary, whichever aroma you prefer, or even one drop of rose if you think it would make it smell nicer for your personal preference, because this will be helping your migraine, which is your first concern.

Another example; let us suppose now that tension is largely responsible for your condition, which in this case is migraine and irregular periods. So we write down all the oils for tension.

'tension: basil, bergamot, camomile, juniper, lavender,

marjoram, melissa, jasmine, neroli, rose, sandalwood and ylang-ylang'

What a long list! If it is only tension you want to treat, then use any one to three oils to make the most relaxing aroma for you. Remember top notes have a sharper aroma, middle notes vary a great deal but are never woody or heavy, base notes are much sweeter and heavier; so decide whether you like a light or a heavy aroma and choose accordingly. We want to treat migraine as well, so write down the oils for that condition which already appear on the tension list, e.g.,

'migraine: basil, camomile, lavender, marjoram, melissa, rose'

If you now turn to irregular periods you will find that camomile, melissa and rose are the oils mentioned there. As these last three oils occur in each ailment, they are the three to use for treatment. If, however, you do not have any rose then lavender or any of the base notes on the tension list could be substituted to obtain the aroma you like.

It is a fascinating occupation choosing and mixing essential oils for use in aromatherapy, and with experience the most effective blend for your particular problem can be worked out. Meanwhile, I will help you with suggested 'recipes' to start you off, and also tell you which oils blend well together for a particular complaint. For pure aroma, on the Table of Essential Oils you will find a list of some other oils with which each blends best. As you know from buying or being given perfumes, certain 'smells' suit some people and not others, so I can only suggest what is acceptable to me. You must find your own end aroma, and the best way of doing that is by trying different combinations of the selected treatment oils.

Any oil can of course be used on its own. In the last example, melissa, rose *or* camomile could be tried if the aroma is pleasing.

For some conditions you will find that it is impossible to arrive at a totally acceptable aroma. So then add a drop or two of any oil which will make the treatment oil acceptable. Jasmine is of particular use here.

No essential oil is 'nice' to take internally, except in tea. Tea made with essential oil is very weak and one can learn to accept the flavour if it means good health, but as there will be at least a thousand combinations, even if you only possess a small selection of oils it should be possible to arrive at a flavour you can enjoy.

Never forget the importance of the attitude of mind in ill-health. Illness is not always completely physical. Remember too, that a small percentage of oil will usually treat a psychological condition whereas a stronger percentage is usually required for a purely physical complaint.

When mixing oils together, neat, for one condition, to be used in a variety of ways, a hypodermic syringe (usually obtainable from your local chemist) is an ideal way of measuring the quantities, and much quicker than counting a lot of drops. But don't forget to put a label on the bottle, and write on it what you have used, for example,

Indigestion		*Indigestion*
2ml peppermint		40 drops peppermint
1ml camomile	or	20 drops camomile
1ml fennel		20 drops fennel

Before giving you the recipes which I have tried (and had success with) on clients, may I remind you that as I said earlier not everyone reacts in the same way to a certain blend, and I have often had to choose an alternative blend for someone where the first did not have the desired effect.

All the recipes will be given in numbers, for use in drops or millilitres. So that when you are mixing a trial amount you can mix in drops to see if it is a successful mix for you, either in your bath or in an oil, or in a tea. For a massage oil trial use 2 teaspoonsful of carrier oil and divide the number of drops given by 4, 5 or 6 (whichever is the easier). I have given the *maximum* number of drops in the recipes as it makes it easier for you to divide into smaller quantities. When you mix your first bottles of massage oil always use the lowest strength — 15 drops; you can always add more if needed. For tea-making, if using more than three oils it is best to omit one, or the tea will be strong. Alternatively, mix a total of around 15 drops and use 12 in your bath and 3 in your tea, or 10 in your bath and 5 in a teaspoonful of carrier oil for massage. But when you find a recipe that suits you, you can then use the numbers for measuring in millilitres using your syringe and making your treatment recipe in a dropper bottle, from which you can use it in any method you like, as follows:

Baths	10-15 drops (also foot and hand baths)
Compress	10 drops in ½ cup water (100ml)
Inhalant	10 drops on paper towel
	10 drops in ½ basin hot water

Massage Oil	15-30 drops in 50ml carrier oil		
Medicine	3-4 drops in red wine or honey and water 2-3 times daily		
Tea	2-3 drops on one tea bag for 3-4 cups of tea, without milk, 3 times daily		

Remember you can decrease the dose for psychological problems and may increase it for physical problems, but at no time have any *one* treatment using more than 10 drops; you may hinder the beneficial effect. You may of course use more than one treatment technique in any one day e.g. drink tea, put oils in the bath *and* use a compress or massage oil.

For the method of using the essential oils in the following recipes turn to the chapters on Simple Aromatherapy Treatment Techniques and Aromatherapy Massage Techniques.

If you would find it more convenient to have oils ready mixed, these can be obtained from the address at the back of this book.

Anti-stretch Marks

	Frankincense	Lavender	Lemongrass
Massage Oil	10	15	5

Arthritis (& Joints)

	Benzoin	Camomile	Rosemary	Sage
Bath	2	2	3	3
Massage Oil	6	6	8	8
Tea	1	1	—	1
	Benzoin	Lavender	Rosemary	Marigold
Bath	1	2	2	3
Massage Oil	4	8	8	12
Tea	—	—	—	2

Arthritis and Rheumatism

	Eucalyptus	Juniper	Marjoram	Rosemary
Bath	2	3	2	3
Massage Oil	6	8	6	8
Tea	—	—	1	1

Bronchitis

	Eucalyptus	Hyssop	Sandalwood
Bath	6	2	2
Compress	6	2	2
Inhalant	6	2	2
Massage Oil	15	10	5
Medicine	2	1	1

Cellulite (& Hangover!)

	Fennel	Juniper	Rosemary	Sage
Bath	4	1	2	2
Massage Oil	12	4	8	8

Chilblains

	Lemon	Marigold
Compress	2	2
Foot bath	5	5
Massage Oil	15	15
Tea	1	1

Cold in the Head

	Basil	Eucalyptus	Peppermint
Bath	4	4	2
Inhalant	4	4	2

Constipation & Cellulite

	Fennel	Rosemary
Bath	5	5
Massage Oil	15	15
Medicine	2	2
Tea	1	1

Cough & Cold

	Benzoin	Bl.Pepper	Eucalyptus	Hyssop
Bath	4	3	4	2
Inhalant	4	2	4	2

Cramp

	Basil	Marjoram	
Bath	5	5	
Massage Oil	15	15	
	Basil	Lemongrass	Marjoram
Bath	6	3	3
Massage Oil	12	8	8

Dermatitis

	Geranium	Juniper	Lavender	Benzoin
Bath	4	2	2	2
Massage Oil	12	6	6	6

Eczema

	Bergamot	Geranium	Juniper	Lavender
Compress	2	2	4	2
Massage Oil	5	5	10	5

High Blood Pressure

	Lavender	Ylang-ylang
Bath	5	5
Massage Oil	15	15
Medicine	2	2
Tea	1	1

Indigestion

	Fennel	Melissa	Peppermint
Medicine	1	1	2
Tea	1	1	1
	Fennel	Peppermint	Sage
Medicine	1	1	1
Tea	1	1	1

Insect Repellent

	Eucalyptus	Peppermint	Cedarwood
Massage Oil	12	6	6

Insomnia

	Camomile	Juniper	Marjoram	Rose
Bath	2	4	4	2
Tea	1	1	—	1

Insomnia & Stress

	Camomile	Juniper	Marjoram	Melissa
Bath	2	4	2	4
Tea	1	1	1	—
	Benzoin	Camomile	Juniper	Neroli
Bath	2	2	2	4
Tea (1)	—	—	—	2
Tea (2)	1	—	—	1

Irregular Periods

	Camomile	Melissa	Rose
Bath	4	4	4
Compress	4	4	4
Massage Oil	10	10	10

Migraine & Rheumatism

	Lavender	Marjoram	Melissa	Sage
Bath	2	2	4	4
Compress	2	2	4	4
Massage Oil	5	5	10	10
Tea	1	1	1	—

Muscular Aches & Pains

	Eucalyptus	Rosemary	Sage
Bath	3	3	4
Compress	3	3	4
Hand/Foot			
Bath	3	3	4
Massage Oil	8	8	12

Muscle Tone

	Bl.Pepper	Lavender	Lemongrass
Bath	4	3	3
Massage Oil	12	8	8

Nervous Tension

	Bergamot	Marjoram	Neroli	Sandal-wood
Bath (1)	—	—	5	—
Bath (2)	2	2	1	2
Massage Oil	4	4	4	4
Tea (1)	1	—	—	1
Tea (2)	—	—	2	—

	Basil	Juniper	Lavender	Ylang-ylang
Bath	1	2	2	1
Massage Oil (1)	4	4	4	4
Massage Oil (2)	—	—	6	12
Tea	—	—	1	1

Perspiring Feet

	Bergamot	Clary sage	Cypress
Foot Bath	4	4	2

Poor Circulation

	Benzoin	Bl.Pepper	Juniper
Bath	2	4	4
Massage Oil	8	12	12
Tea	1	1	1

Sinus Problems

	Basil	Eucalyptus	Lavender	Peppermint
Bath	3	3	3	3
Inhalant	3	3	3	3
Massage Oil	8	8	8	8

Tonic for Hair

Cedarwood	Juniper	Rosemary
10	10	15

Use in 50ml surgical spirit, not carrier oil

11.

Table of Essential Oils

How pure is an essential oil?
This is not an easy question to answer, because the production is not necessarily a simple procedure. Some plants yield essential oil in a straightforward manner, such as steam distillation and expression, as we have already seen in the chapter on Essential Oils. With other plants and with the gums from trees it is a more complicated process, using a volatile solvent in a closed apparatus and a vacuum still, which yields a solid consisting of the essential 'oil' and natural waxes and colour. This substance is called a *concrete*, which is then mixed with alcohol to remove the waxes, and this leaves an *absolute*, usually thicker liquids than oils obtained by distillation. These absolutes are, of course, very expensive and have a really superb aroma.

To give an idea of the complexity, let us take Rose as an example.

Rose absolute is produced (sometimes called Rese-de-Grasse or Rose-de-Mai) in some countries, and this is ususally a browny-yellow colour. Other countries produce a Rose Otto (or Attar of Roses) which is obtained by steam distillation and is much clearer, almost colourless. This can be even more expensive than a Rose absolute, but Rose Otto is thought to be the best therapeutically, though the aroma is perhaps a little less exotic.

Absolute oils, if not produced skilfully, often have left in them some of the alcohol used in their production; this can be detected in the aroma by a skilled 'nose'★ and counts as an adulterated oil.

Attar of Roses may also be skilfully adulterated either in the country of origin or elsewhere by the addition of inferior natural rose oils or by synthetic materials, and buyers in this country must exercise great care when purchasing these oils.
Pomades are made by the process of enfleurage. This is when

★'nose' is the official name given to a perfumer of 20 or more years experience in smelling essential oils.

layers of fat are covered with fresh flowers, which are topped up until the fat is fully charged with the flower perfume. After leaving for several days, the flowers are strained off and the resultant waxy substance is called a pomade. The essential oil can then be extracted from the fat by means of a solvent, and once more the purity of that oil is dependent on how well the solvent is evaporated from the essential oil.

Blends can be made from various pure and natural oils mixed together (i.e. the neat essential oils you will mix for yourself for baths or teas are *blends*). However, in the trade, a blend is an adulterated oil, as it is always sold under *one* name, even though two different oils may be in the container. For example, if a producer of rosemary oil has a poor crop of rosemary, he can adulterate it by adding camphor oil, which will give the poor rosemary a better 'rosemary' aroma.

Blends can also consist of synthetic materials mixed in with the pure oil, giving a good aroma but making the cost substantially cheaper.

So you can see that *blended* oils while often quite suitable for the perfumery trade, do not have the correct therapeutic qualities we need for aromatherapy, and therefore cannot be classed as pure essential oils by an aromatherapist.

Being natural products, the quantity, quality and therefore the properties of essential oils vary from season to season with weather conditions, etc., as I have already said earlier in the book, so the price varies accordingly with each harvest. Price also varies with the amount of oil found in a plant; for example, eucalyptus is rich in oil but jasmine, rose and orange blossom contain only a little. Therefore you must expect to pay up to *ten or twelve* times as much for these three oils as for most other oils, because much larger quantities of petals are required to yield a given amount of oil, and much more work is involved. It is possible to buy in stores and some herbal shops jasmine and other oils which are diluted in some form, either with alcohol or carrier oil. The bottle will not state that it has been diluted, but the price should tell you! This means you could use it as a 'ready mixed' oil but it could not be used in the recipes given in this book, all of which require undilute, unblended pure essential oils.

Selecting an essential oil for therapeutic use is full of traps for the unwary or inexperienced, and the wisest course of action is to obtain supplies only from an honest, reliable source in whom you can trust. This element of trust is most important in the essential oil business, as the selection of pure oils is very much an art, combined with knowledge and wide experience.

TABLE OF ESSENTIAL OILS

Alphabetical List of Oils

Name	Note	General Effect
Basil	Top	Uplifting and refreshing
Benzoin	Base	Warming and relaxing
Bergamot	Top	Uplifting and refreshing; also relaxing
Black Pepper	Middle	Stimulating
Calendula (Marigold)	Base	Healing and rejuvenating
Camomile	Middle	Refreshing and relaxing
Camphor	Base	Cooling and stimulating
Cedarwood	Base	Sedative
Clary Sage	Top to Middle	Warming and relaxing (aphrodisiac)
Cypress	Middle to Base	Relaxing and refreshing
Eucalyptus	Top	Head clearing
Fennel	Middle	Carminative (eases wind and stomach pains)
Frankincense	Base	Relaxing and rejuvenating
Geranium	Middle	Refreshing and relaxing
Hyssop	Middle	Decongestant (respiratory)
Jasmine	Base	Relaxing and soothing
Juniper	Middle	Refreshing, stimulating and relaxing
Lavender	Middle	Refreshing, relaxing, generally therapeutic
Lemon	Top	Refreshing and stimulating
Lemongrass	Top	Toning and refreshing
Marjoram	Middle	Warming and fortifying
Melissa	Middle	Uplifting and refreshing
Myrrh	Base	Cooling and toning
Neroli (Orange blossom)	Base	Ultra-relaxing
Patchouli	Base	Relaxing
Peppermint	Middle to Top	Cooling and refreshing
Pine Needle	Middle to Base	Refreshing and antiseptic
Rose	Base	Relaxing and soothing
Rosemary	Middle	Invigorating and refreshing
Sage	Top	Decongestant (circulatory)

Name	Note	General Effect
Sandalwood	Base	Relaxing
Thyme	Top to Middle	Antiseptic
Ylang-Ylang	Base	Relaxing

TOP NOTES

These are all stimulating and uplifting.

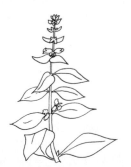

BASIL
Blends well with:
  bergamot
  geranium
  hyssop

There are many varieties of sweet basil, which originated in Asia and was extensively used in Indian medicine. More often grown now in Reunion, France, Cyprus, Seychelles. The flowering tops and leaves are used and extraction is by distillation. The leaves are heart-shaped, and are a love symbol in Italy. It is an oil which clears the head and is uplifting — it makes a good nerve tonic.

Digestive: indigestion, vomiting, intestinal infections, gastro-enteritis

Head: earache, colds, sinus, migraine

Muscular: spasm

Nervous: anxiety, depression, hysteria, indecision, nervous debility, tonic

Respiratory: asthma, bronchitis, catarrh, hiccups

Skin: sluggish or congested, insect repellant, soothes wasp stings (use neat)

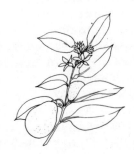

BERGAMOT
Blends well with:
  cypress
  jasmine
  lavender
  neroli

Bergamot belongs to the citrus family. The oil is obtained by expression from the fresh peel of the fruit of Citrus Bergamia after the juice has been extracted. The main production area is Southern Italy. The trees grow to a height of 15 feet (4.5m), and fruits are picked December to February. The small round fruits change from green to yellow and the newly ripe fruits give the best oil. The yield is half a kilo from 100 kilos of fruits and the colour should be yellowish to browny green. It is used prominently in Eau-de-Cologne and lavender water. Bergamot oil is liable to skilful adulteration. It is a powerful antiseptic and is excellent (personal experience) for cold sores (herpes), and is also helpful when used in the bath in the case of vaginal pruritis. The leaves of the plant are used in the manufacture of Earl Grey tea.

    Cancer: preventative, and treatment
    Digestive: colic, flatulence, gastro-enteritis, indigestion
    Excretory: cystitis, urinary infections
    Head: bad breath, deodorizer, sore throat, tonsillitis
    Nervous: anxiety, depression
    Respiratory: bronchitis (especially when used with lemon oil)
    Skin: acne, oily, seborrhoea of scalp, herpes, psoriasis, ulcers,
        wounds

Note: Do not use indiscriminately on skin, and never neat, as pigmentation can occur. Bergamot increases photo-sensitivity of skin, therefore used in sun tan preparations

CLARY SAGE
Blends well with:
    cedarwood
    citrus oils
    frankincense
    geranium
    jasmine
    juniper
    lavender
    sandalwood

Russia has the largest output of clary sage oil, though small amounts are produced in Morocco and the South of France. It has high fixative power and flowering tops and foliage of Salvia Sclarea are used. The word Clary originates from the Latin for clear, because an eye lotion used to be made from the seeds of this plant. Dry soil, high elevation, shade from olive trees, sun and *spring* rain, give a much superior oil than that from rich moist soil at low levels. Quality also varies according to use of manure, the time of day of picking, the dryness of the plant, and whether the seeds are completely formed. Known in Germany as Muscatel sage; together with elder flowers it was used in the making of German 'Muscatel' wines. Used by the Italians in various brands of vermouth. Now an invaluable ingredient of best Eau-de-Colognes and lavender water.

Circulatory: high blood pressure
Head: sore throat
Menstrual: irregularity, painful
Nervous: depression (good nerve tonic)
Skin: inflamed, mature

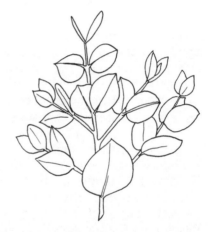

EUCALYPTUS
Blends well with:
  benzoin
  lavender
  pine

This oil is obtained from the fresh leaves which are rich in essential oil. Although eucalyptus is one of the tallest trees in the world, trees are kept beheaded to make branches more accessible. Grown in Australia, Tasmania, Algeria, France. There are about 200 species of eucalyptus. Has been used to rub countless chests over the years, to improve breathing in colds and sinusitis, and has a definite cooling effect on body temperature — a febrifuge.

Digestive: diarrhoea
Excretory: cystitis, diuretic
Head: colds, congestive headache, sinus, throat infections
Muscular: aches and pains, rheumatoid arthritis
Nervous: neuralgia
Obesity: fluid retention
Respiratory: asthma, bronchitis, catarrh, coughs
Skin: good antiseptic, herpes, ulcers, wounds

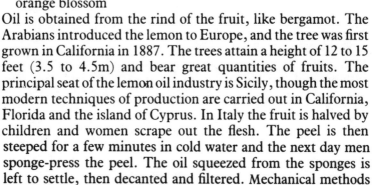

LEMON

Blends well with:
  lavender
  orange blossom

Oil is obtained from the rind of the fruit, like bergamot. The Arabians introduced the lemon to Europe, and the tree was first grown in California in 1887. The trees attain a height of 12 to 15 feet (3.5 to 4.5m) and bear great quantities of fruits. The principal seat of the lemon oil industry is Sicily, though the most modern techniques of production are carried out in California, Florida and the island of Cyprus. In Italy the fruit is halved by children and women scrape out the flesh. The peel is then steeped for a few minutes in cold water and the next day men sponge-press the peel. The oil squeezed from the sponges is left to settle, then decanted and filtered. Mechanical methods are also used, but the hand processed oil is the better quality.

  Circulatory: anaemia, chilblains, poor circulation, varicose veins, high blood pressure
  Digestive: diabetes, vomiting
  Excretory: kidneys
  Head: conjunctivitis, laryngitis, mouth ulcers
  Muscular: arthritis, rheumatism
  Obesity: congestion in tissues
  Respiratory: asthma, catarrh, colds, 'flu
  Skin: boils, broken capillaries, greasy skin, herpes, insect bites, mouth ulcers, wrinkles

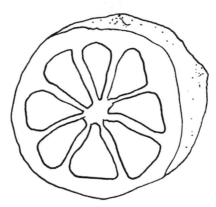

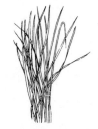

LEMONGRASS
Blends well with:
  geranium
  jasmine
  lavender

Lemongrass oil is obtained by distillation from two species of grasses which grow wild and are also cultivated in Madras, Malay, West Indies. Distillation takes place from July to January and about 350 kilos of grass is needed to yield 20ml of oil. It is one of the largest production essential oils — over 2000 tons a year being distilled. The oil is the colour of dry sherry and has a lemonish smell which is quite powerful.

  Digestive: colitis, indigestion, gastro-enteritis
  Muscular: poor tone, slack tissue
  Skin: acne and open pores, tonic

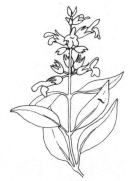

SAGE
Blends well with:
  bergamot
  hyssop
  lemon
  lavender
  rosemary

From leaves which are dried in the hot sun before distilling. It is comparatively expensive because of the hard labour involved in preparation. The herb is indigenous to the countries bordering the northern coasts of the Mediterranean. It is a yellow oil with a camphor-like smell. Sometimes used to adulterate rosemary and spike lavender oils. Sage tea, regularly taken for four weeks before childbirth, relieves labour pains.

  Excretory: diuretic
  Muscular: all rheumatic conditions, aches and pains in joints
  Nervous: good nerve tonic
  Obesity: congestion, fluid retention
  Skin: sluggish or congested, ulcers, wounds, tonic

MIDDLE NOTES

These affect most body systems and general metabolism.

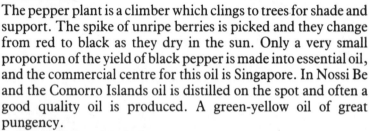

BLACK PEPPER
Blends well with:
  frankincense
  sandalwood

The pepper plant is a climber which clings to trees for shade and support. The spike of unripe berries is picked and they change from red to black as they dry in the sun. Only a very small proportion of the yield of black pepper is made into essential oil, and the commercial centre for this oil is Singapore. In Nossi Be and the Comorro Islands oil is distilled on the spot and often a good quality oil is produced. A green-yellow oil of great pungency.

  Circulatory: stimulating
  Digestive: colic, constipation, food poisoning, indigestion, loss of appetite
  Excretory: pain, burning, stimulates urination (diuretic)
  Head: colds, headache caused by cold in head, toothache
  Muscular: aches and pains, externally analgesic, lack of tone
  Respiratory: catarrh, coughs

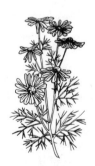

CAMOMILE
Blends well with:
  geranium
  lavender
  patchouli
  rose

Roman camomile is distilled from the dried flowers of Anthemis Nobilis. Used a lot because of its Azulene content which is not present in flower but forms as the essential oil is distilled out of the plant. Camomile changes with exposure to light and air from blue to browny-yellow. Roman camomile produced in Belgium is light blue-green-yellowy brown. In England the centre for this oil is Long Melford. German camomile (from Germany, Hungary, Russia) is deep blue and contains more azulene. It is distilled from Matricaria Chamomilla. This oil covers most disorders and has very low toxicity, therefore is very useful for children. Used in hair shampoo to help to lighten the hair. Moroccan Camomile is obtained from Osmanis Mixta.

Digestive: diarrhoea, flatulence, gastritis, indigestion (especially in children), liver disorders, loss of appetite, peptic ulcers, stomach ulcers

Head: conjunctivitis, earache, teething, toothache

Menstrual: haemorrhage, irregularity, irritation, menopause, painful

Muscular: all aches and pains — especially after sport, arthritis and rheumatism

Nervous: anxiety, depression, hysteria, insomnia, irritability, neuralgia, tantrums (in children), tonic

Skin: acne, anti-allergic, antiseptic, broken veins, burns, dermatitis, dryness, hyper-sensitivity, inflammation, irritability, wounds

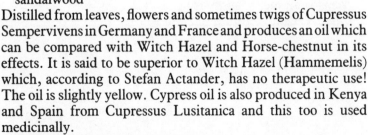

CYPRESS
Blends well with:
juniper
pine
sandalwood

Distilled from leaves, flowers and sometimes twigs of Cupressus Sempervivens in Germany and France and produces an oil which can be compared with Witch Hazel and Horse-chestnut in its effects. It is said to be superior to Witch Hazel (Hammemelis) which, according to Stefan Actander, has no therapeutic use! The oil is slightly yellow. Cypress oil is also produced in Kenya and Spain from Cupressus Lusitanica and this too is used medicinally.

Cancer: prevention and treatment
Circulatory: sluggish

Digestive: diarrhoea
Excretory: haemorrhoids
Head: laryngitis, nose bleed
Menstrual: haemorrhage, excessive loss, menopause, ovary
                problems, painful
Muscular: cramp
Nervous: calmative, irritability
Respiratory: asthma, spasmodic cough
Skin: oily, broken capillaries, mature, sweating, tonic,
      varicose veins

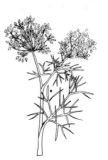

FENNEL
Blends well with:
  geranium
  lavender
  rose
  sandalwood

There is a sweet fennel oil and a bitter fennel oil distilled from the
crushed seeds. Fennel is widely grown throughout the world —
the Mediterranean, India, Asia, America and Europe. It has a
pleasant sweet aroma reminiscent of aniseed, and is traditionally
used in cooking. Because of its effect on the hormones, and its
diuretic qualities, it is an invaluable oil for reducing obesity. It is
also well known for its aid to digestive problems (used in
gripewater for babies).

Digestive: colic, colitis, constipation, flatulence, food poison-
                ing, hiccough, nausea, vomiting
Excretory: diuretic, kidney stones
Head: weak eyesight
Menstrual: menopausal irregularities
Obesity: cellulite, fluid retention

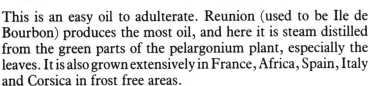

GERANIUM
Blends well with nearly all oils, especially:
   basil
   citrus oils
   rose

This is an easy oil to adulterate. Reunion (used to be Ile de Bourbon) produces the most oil, and here it is steam distilled from the green parts of the pelargonium plant, especially the leaves. It is also grown extensively in France, Africa, Spain, Italy and Corsica in frost free areas.
   Digestive: diarrhoea, gastro-enteritis
   Excretory: mild diuretic, stones, urinary tract disorders
   Head: throat and mouth infections
   Menstrual: menopausal haemorrhage, leucorrhoea, sterility
   Nervous: anxiety, depression, neuralgia
   Obesity: congestion, fluid retention
   Skin: cleansing, dermatitis, dry eczema, inflamed, oily, sluggish, tonic, ulcers, wounds

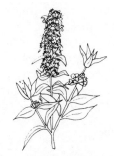

HYSSOP
Blends well with:
   citrus oils
   clary sage
   lavender
   rosemary
   sage

Hyssop is well known for its medicinal uses, and is excellent as a tonic. The oil is obtained from cultivated plants in Provence and Germany, and is often used in Eau-de-Cologne. The Hebrews called this plant Ezob and our name for hyssop stems from this: 'Purge me with hyssop and I shall be clean', Psalm 51:9. It is especially good for asthma and related problems, in fact any respiratory problem. It is a small plant with thin leaves and small blue flowers, both of which are used in distillation to obtain essential oil (People prone to epilepsy should not take hyssop except in homeopathic doses.)

Circulatory: normalizing, e.g. raises and lowers blood
          pressure
Digestive: flatulence, loss of appetite, mild laxative, gastro-
          enteritis
Excretory: kidney stones
Menstrual: leucorrhoea, scanty
Nervous: calmative, general debility
Respiratory: asthma, bronchitis, catarrh, coughs, hay fever,
          emphysema
Skin: bruises, eczema, wounds

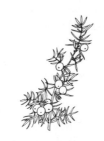

JUNIPER
Blends well with:
  benzoin
  cypress
  lavender
  sandalwood
Juniper oil is distilled from the dried fruits of the juniper bush
which grows in Europe and Canada. The oil is colourless or pale
yellow and grows darker and thicker with age and exposure to
air. Used to flavour gin. Known since ancient times for its
antiseptic and diuretic qualities, and is very useful in worried or
anxious states of mind.
  Circulatory: stimulating
  Digestive: colic, flatulence, indigestion
  Excretory: cystitis, diuretic, fluid retention, haemorrhoids
  Menstrual: leucorrhoea, painful, scanty
  Muscular: rheumatic pain
  Nervous: anxiety, calmative, insomnia, stress, tonic
  Skin: acne, oily, eczema, dermatitis, seborrhoea of scalp,
          tonic

LAVENDER
Blends well with most oils, especially:
  citrus oils
  clary sage
  patchouli
  pine
  rosemary

This oil is the most used and most versatile of all the essential oils. It is distilled from Lavandula Vera which is native to the Alpine slopes of the Mediterranean. The oil is obtained from wild plants in France, and cultivated plants in England and Tasmania. Oil glands are embedded among tiny star shaped hairs with which the flowers, leaves and stems are covered, and the aroma has a comparatively short life. Used to be subject to extensive adulteration, but now lavandin and spike lavender are used instead of lavender in soaps, household goods and cheaper perfumes, leaving lavender for therapeutic use and the better quality perfumes. It is a very useful oil (like camomile) especially when symptoms are due to a nervous problem. Generally it acts best in conjunction with another oil:

Circulatory: lowers high blood pressure, lymphatic congestion

Digestive: colic, flatulence, gastro-enteritis, indigestion, nausea

Excretory: cystitis

Head: bad breath, conjunctivitis, earache, headache, migraine, nose and throat infections

Menstrual: irregularity, leucorrhoea, scanty

Muscular: aches and pains, rheumatism, sprains

Nervous: anxiety, depression, general debility, irritability, palpitations

Obesity: cellulite, fluid retention

Respiratory: all catarrhal complaints, flu

Skin: acne rosacea, all types, alopecia, bites, boils, burns, dermatitis, eczema, inflammation, insect bites, psoriasis, rejunvenative, sunburn

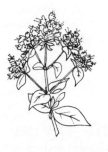

MARJORAM
Blends well with:
  bergamot
  lavender
  rosemary

Distilled from the flowering heads of sweet marjoram, Origanum Majorana. The plant grows in Spain, Southern France and Tunisia. It was grown and used in ancient times by the Egyptians. The oil is colourless with a persistent odour. A

very 'comforting' oil if low in spirits.
Circulatory: lowers high blood pressure
Digestive: constipation, relieves spasm in intestines
Head: colds in the head, headache, migraine
Menstrual: leucorrhoea, painful
Muscular: all muscular pain, bruises, neuralgia, spasm, sprains, strains
Nervous: anxiety, calmative, general debility, insomnia, irritability
Respiratory: asthma, catarrh

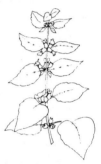

MELISSA
Blends well with:
geranium
lavender
neroli
ylang-ylang

The local name in Southern Europe is 'heart's delight', and it is often called the 'elixir of life'. It has been used medicinally since the seventeeth century, and is a very cheering oil, making a good general tonic. It is also known as balm oil, and is obtained by distilling the leaves and tops of Melissa officinalis, which is native to Mediterranean countries and is cultivated in the U.S.A.
Digestive: flatulence, indigestion, nausea
Head: headache, migraine, temperature
Menstrual: irregular, painful, sterility
Nervous: hysteria, lowers high blood pressure, shock, tension, tonic
Skin: bee and wasp stings

PEPPERMINT
Blends well with:
benzoin
rosemary

Oil is distilled from the leaves and flowering tops of Mentha cultivated in Europe, U.S.A. and Japan. English oil is reputed to be the best. It is widely used in confectionery and toiletry as well as being an excellent therapeutic oil. Use internally instead of aspirin — much healthier for your stomach.

Digestive: diarrhoea, flatulence, gall stones, indigestion, stomach pain, travel sickness

Head: bad breath, colds, headache, migraine (digestive origin), sinusitis

Menstrual: irregular, painful, scanty

Nervous: general debility, neuralgia, shock

Respiratory: bronchitis, catarrh, coughs, flu

Skin: inflammation, insect repellant, irritation, toxic congestion

PINE NEEDLE

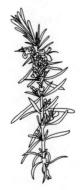

Blends well with:
cedarwood
rosemary
sage

Distilled from the needles and cones of several species of conifer. Good oils are obtained from North East Russia and the Austrian Tyrol. Used extensively in soaps, bath preparations and, because of its antiseptic qualities, in detergents, etc.

Digestive: gall stones

Excretory: cystitis, kidneys

Head: sinus

Nervous: general debility

Respiratory: all infections of respiratory tract, asthma, bronchitis, flu

ROSEMARY

Blends well with:
basil
cedarwood
citrus oils
frankincense
lavender
peppermint

Distilled from the flowering tops and leaves of Rosmarinus officinalis, grown in countries bordering the Mediterranean but chiefly Southern France, Spain, and the Dalmatian Islands. (garden legend has it that 'where rosemary thrives the mistress is master') Mostly made in Spain, where the quality varies from very high to very low. Oil of the most consistently high quality comes from Tunisia. It is possible to adulterate rosemary oil with turpentine, sage and spike oils. The pure oil is used in Eau-de-Cologne. It has been in therapeutic use for hundreds of years.

Circulatory: lymphatic congestion

Digestive: colitis, constipation, diarrhoea, flatulence, gall stones, gastro-enteritis, stomach pains

Excretory: diuretic

Head: headache, mental fatigue, migraine, stengthens memory

Menstrual: lack of periods, leucorrhoea

Muscular: aches and pains, arthritis, rheumatism

Nervous: general debility, loss of nerve function, e.g., epilepsy, paralysis, mental strain

Obesity: fluid retention

Respiratory: asthma, chronic bronchitis, coughs, flu

Skin: alopecia, cleansing, dandruff, scalp disorders, stimulating, wounds

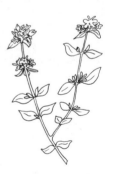

THYME

Blends well with:
   bergamot
   lemon
   melissa
   rosemary

The oil is obtained from flowering tops by steam distillation. Like lavender, thyme has many therapeutic qualities, and it is used extensively in cooking as well as in medicine. It is a stong antiseptic and gives protection against colds and flu; it is also a good nerve tonic. Thyme is said to stimulate the production of white corpuscles in the blood in infectious diseases. Thyme and rosemary oils in tea are excellent for headaches and nervous problems.

Circulatory: stimulating, low blood pressure

Digestive: sluggish, flatulence
Excretory: diuretic
Head: colds, flu, headaches, sinusitis, sore throats, tonsillitis
Menstrual: irregularity, abnormal cessation, leucorrhoea
Muscular: rheumatism, arthritis
Nervous: insomnia, anxiety, nervous debility, depression
Respiratory: catarrh, coughs, whooping cough, bronchitis,
emphysema, asthma
Skin: boils, sores, hair loss

BASE NOTES

All base notes are sedative.

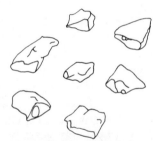

BENZOIN
Blends well with:
rose
sandalwood

Exuded resin of benzoin.

Benzoin is collected as a resin exuded from the trunk after the bark is cut, and is in solid brown to white brittle pieces. More processing is required to bring the benzoin to liquid form. Benzoin comes from trees native to Thailand and Sumatra, and is an ingredient of incense. Commonly known as 'friar's balsam'.

Circulatory: stimulating
Excretory: cystitis, discharges
Joints: rheumatoid arthritis, gout
Nervous: emotional exhaustion, tension
Respiratory: asthma, bronchitis, coughs, flu
Skin: cracked, dry, dermatitis, irritable, wounds

CAMPHOR
Blends well with:
frankincense

Camphor is a solid substance which, together with the essential oil, is present in the wood of the camphor tree (Cinnamomum camphora) which grows naturally in China and Japan, and is cultivated in Sri Lanka and California. Mostly used in the production of celluloid.

Digestive: constipation, flatulence, gastro-enteritis
Excretory: diuretic
Nervous: depression, general debility, insomnia, shock
Respiratory: as an ingredient for inhaling
Skin: acne, bruises, burns, oily, rheumatic inflammation, ulcers, wounds

CEDARWOOD
Blends well with:
  bergamot
  cypress
  jasmine
  juniper
  neroli
  rosemary

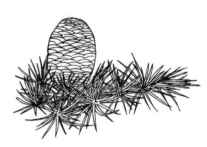

One of the earliest essential oils, used in the preservation of mummies, cedarwood is obtained by steam distillation from the wood of Cedrus atlantica which grows in North Africa. It has been used for many years by natives for medicinal purposes.

Excretory: cystitis, difficulty or pain
Nervous: chronic anxiety states
Skin: acne, oily, alopecia, dandruff, seborrhoea of scalp, insect repellant, irritation
Respiratory: bronchitis, catarrh, coughs

FRANKINCENSE
(*olibanum*)
Blends well with:
  basil
  black pepper
  camphor
  citrus oils
  geranium
  lavender
  pine
  sandalwood

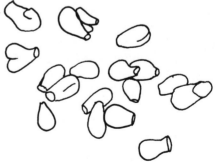

'Tears' of Frankincense.

Frankincense is a whitish gum which has to be dissolved and

distilled to produce essential oil. The trees grow in East Africa and the aromatic resin permeates the bark. (Used in Egyptian times in rejuvenating face masks.) This, with myrrh, was first used as incense and is produced mainly in Iran and Lebanon. Was once highly valuable, hence offering to baby Jesus.

Excretory: cystitis, haemorrhoids
Nervous: anxiety, tension
Respiratory: catarrh and other mucous conditions
Skin: inflamed, poor tonicity, rejuvenative, ulcers, wounds

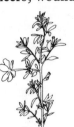

JASMINE
Blends well with all oils, especially
    citrus oils

Obtained by means of solvents or enfleurage from the flowers of Jasminum grandiflorum. The best absolute is extracted by means of the solvent ether and, although expensive, much *less* is needed to give the desired effect; therefore it is economical in use and should be used where the aroma is important. It is most effective on the nervous system, and is invaluable for symptoms with a psychological and psychosomatic origin.

Menstrual: childbirth, pain of any kind, uterine disorders
Nervous: apathy, depression, listlessness, nervous debility,
    sedative and uplifting
Respiratory: breathing difficulties, bronchial spasm, catarrh,
    cough, hoarseness
Skin: all types, especially dry, irritable, sensitive, dermatitis
    (in a depressed condition)

MARIGOLD
(*Calendula*)
Blends well with:
    citrus oils
    geranium
    juniper
    lavender
    pine needle
    sandalwood

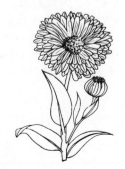

Calendula is of Egyptian origin, valued as a medicinal plant. Excellent for reducing inflammation (e.g. chilblains and rheumatic inflammation) and renewing body tissue. The petals (containing carotene) are used for this oil, and the petals can be chopped up and used in a salad or cooked with rice to colour it yellow, instead of using saffron.

Circulatory: chilblains, haemorrhoids, inflammation, varicose veins

Digestive: enteritis, gall bladder problems, gastritis, indigestion, liver congestion, stomach ulcers

Menstrual: irregular, menopause, painful

Muscular: rheumatism, arthritis

Nervous: anxiety, nervous disorders

Skin: bruises, burns, chilblains, inflammation, rejuvenation, skin diseases, sprains, ulcers, wounds

Gum of Myrrh.

MYRRH

Blends well with:
  camphor
  lavender

Myrrh is a gum resin which naturally exudes from the trunk of Commiphora myrrha, and is then distilled for the essential oil. Used in rejuvenating face masks during Egyptian times, and also for embalming. Mentioned in ancient history (about 1700 BC). When Joseph was sold by his brothers to the Ishmaelite caravan, their camels were carrying gum, balm and myrrh to Egypt.

Digestive: diarrhoea, flatulence, loss of appetite

Excretory: haemorroids

Head: bad breath, mouth ulcers, pyorrhoea, thrush

Respiratory: all types of discharges, soothes respiratory tract

Skin: cooling, anti-inflammatory, rejuvenative, ulcers, wounds

ORANGE BLOSSOM
(*Neroli*)

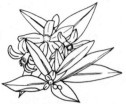

Blends well with most oils, expecially:
  benzoin
  clary sage
  geranium
  lavender

Often called 'neroli', perhaps because the wife of a famous prince in Nerola, Italy, used it to perfume her bath water and her gloves. It is the oil distilled from the fresh blossoms of bitter orange, oil of Neroli Bigarade. (The oil distilled from sweet orange, oil of Neroli Portugal, is not so useful.) A luxury oil used mainly for its aroma, it is a very effective anti-depressant. It is distilled mostly in Southern France, a pale yellow oil indispensible in the making of good quality Eau-de-Colognes, and orange flower water is a by-product of distillation. The best oils come from France and Tunisia, and although expensive, like jasmine, it has a tenacious aroma and is economical in use.

  Digestive: chronic diarrhoea (due to stress), flatulence
  Nervous: anxiety, calmative, depression, fear, hysteria, insomnia, palpitations, panic, shock
  Skin: all types, especially dry, broken capillaries, irritable, regenerative

PATCHOULI

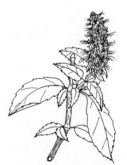

Blends well with:
  bergamot
  geranium
  lavender
  myrrh
  neroli
  pine needle
  rose

Obtained from young leaves cut whenever five are growing on one stem at any one time, and dried before being steam distilled. No more oil is present in older leaves. Interesting in that small quantities will uplift but larger doses sedate. Probably originated in the Philippine Islands, but the main supply now comes from Indonesia, mostly distilled in Singapore.

  Obesity: fluid retention
  Nervous: anxiety, depression
  Skin: heals cracked skin, dries weeping sores and wounds

ROSE
Blends well with:
  bergamot
  clary sage
  geranium
  jasmine
  patchouli
  sandalwood
  and many more

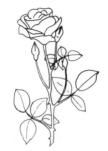

Obtained from the flowers Rosa Centifolia by means of volatile solvents. Bulgarian Rose Otto distilled from Rosa Damascena is the best oil, but Morocco is the largest producer. In France the production of rose oil is very small, and is in fact a by-product from the making of rose water, when the essential oil floats on the top. Of the three superbly aromatic oils, rose oil has the most uses. Like jasmine and neroli, although expensive, very little is needed, and it should be used where the aroma is of importance. It is the least toxic essence and can therefore be used on children.

Circulatory: poor blood circulation

Digestive: constipation, liver problems, peptic ulcer (due to stress), nausea, vomiting, weak stomach

Head: conjunctivitis, earache, headache

Menstrual: impurities in womb, irregularity, leucorrhoea, sterility

Nervous: depression, insomnia, nervous tension, stress

Skin: antiseptic, all types, especially dry, inflamed, mature, sensitive

SANDALWOOD
Blends well with:
  benzoin
  black pepper
  cypress
  frankincense
  neroli
  ylang-ylang

heartwood

The best oil comes from Mysore in East India. The evergreen trees are not cut down until fully mature and showing signs of dying. The oil is in the heartwood at the centre of the tree (not in the bark) and the roots. The heartwood takes 30 years to become 3 inches (7cm) in diameter, and the oil is obtained by steam distillation. The best trees are used for wood for cabinet making.

Digestive: colic, diarrhoea, gastritis, hiccups, nausea, vomiting

Nervous: depression, tension

Respiratory: catarrh, cough, hiccups, laryngitis, sore throat

Skin: dry, inflamed, irritable

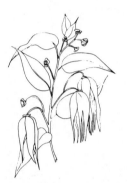

YLANG-YLANG
Blends well with most oils, especially:
jasmine
sandalwood

Obtained by distillation from the flowers of Cananga odorata (the name means 'flower of flowers'). The best plants are grown in the Philippines and Reunion. In Manila the tree blossoms all the year round, but the best flowers for oil are picked in May and June only, early in the morning. Ylang-ylang is much used in high class perfumery, and often called the poor man's jasmine. Many different qualities of oil are available and oil from Javanese trees of the same name is decidedly inferior, probably due to climatic and soil conditions. Dry soil, high elevation, shade from olive trees and *spring* rain give a much superior oil than that from rich moist soil at low levels.

Circulation: high blood pressure

Digestive: gastro-enteritis

Nervous: depression, insomnia, tension

Skin: oily

12.

Therapeutic Cross Reference

Problem	Top Notes	Middle Notes	Base Notes
Circulation			
anaemia	lemon thyme	camomile	
chilblains	lemon		marigold
haemorrhoids (piles)			frankincense marigold myrrh
high blood pressure	clary sage lemon	cypress juniper	ylang-ylang
low blood pressure	sage thyme	lavender marjoram melissa	
poor circulation	lemon	hyssop rosemary	
		black pepper cypress juniper	benzoin rose
		rosemary	
sluggish lymph	sage	lavender rosemary	
varicose veins	lemon	cypress	marigold
Digestive			
bilious attack		peppermint	
colic	bergamot	black pepper	sandalwood fennel hyssop
		juniper lavender peppermint	
colitis, enteritis	lemongrass thyme	lavender rosemary	marigold
constipation		black pepper fennel hyssop	camphor
		marjoram rosemary	
diabetes	eucalyptus lemon	geranium juniper rosemary	
diarrhoea	eucalyptus sage	camomile cypress geranium	myrrh sandalwood
		juniper lavender peppermint	
		rosemary	

Problem	Top Notes	Middle Notes	Base Notes
flatulence	basil bergamot sage	*fennel* hyssop juniper lavender melissa *peppermint* rosemary	camphor myrrh
food poisoning	bergamot eucalyptus *lemon*	black pepper fennel	
gall stones	basil bergamot *lemongrass* thyme	peppermint rosemary *pine*	camphor marigold ylang-ylang
gastro enteritis		camomile geranium hyssop *lavender* rosemary	
heartburn		black pepper	
indigestion (dyspepsia)	basil *bergamot* lemongrass *sage* thyme	black pepper *camomile fennel* hyssop juniper lavender melissa *peppermint rosemary*	marigold
liver	lemon sage	peppermint rosemary	marigold rose
liver (cirrhosis)		juniper rosemary	myrrh
loss of appetite	bergamot	black pepper camomile fennel hyssop juniper	
nausea		fennel lavender melissa	rose sandalwood
stomach pains	*bergamot*	peppermint *camomile fennel lavender*	
stomach ulcers	lemon	*peppermint* rosemary	marigold rose
travel sickness		camomile geranium	
vomiting	lemon	peppermint fennel peppermint	rose

Problem	Top Notes	Middle Notes	Base Notes
Excretory			
cystitis	bergamot eucalyptus sage	black pepper fennel juniper lavender pine	benzoin
diuretics		cypress *fennel* hyssop juniper rosemary	frankincense sandalwood
kidneys (general)	eucalyptus lemon sage *thyme*	fennel geranium *juniper* lavender pine	camphor sandalwood
stones	lemon	fennel geranium hyssop juniper	cedarwood sandalwood
Head			
bad breath	bergamot thyme	lavender peppermint rosemary	myrrh
colds	basil eucalyptus lemon	black pepper marjoram melissa peppermint rosemary	benzoin
conjunctivitis	lemon	*camomile* geranium lavender	rose
ear ache	basil	camomile hyssop lavender	rose
headache	lemon eucalyptus (congestive headaches)	*camomile* lavender (digestive headaches) peppermint	
laryngitis	lemon sage thyme	cypress	frankincense sandalwood
migraine	basil eucalyptus (congestive)	*camomile lavender marjoram* melissa *peppermint* (digestive) rosemary	rose

Problem	Top Notes	Middle Notes	Base Notes
mouth wash (gum strengthener)	lemon	camomile	myrrh
nose bleed	sage	fennel	frankincense
sinus	*basil* eucalyptus lemon	cypress	
sore throat	bergamot clary sage	lavender peppermint pine	sandalwood
	eucalyptus lemon sage	geranium lavender	
teething		camomile	
toothache	sage	black pepper juniper	
		peppermint	
weak sight		fennel rosemary	
Menstrual			
haemorrhage	*sage*	camomile *cypress* geranium	frankincense rose
		juniper	
irregularity	basil *sage*	camomile clary sage *fennel*	marigold rose
		lavender *melissa* peppermint	
lack of periods	clary sage *sage* thyme	*camomile* fennel hyssop	rose
		melissa	
leucorrhoea	bergamot eucalyptus	geranium hyssop juniper	frankincense myrrh
		lavender marjoram	
		rosemary	
menopause	*sage*	camomile *cypress* fennel	marigold
		geranium	

Problem	Top Notes	Middle Notes	Base Notes
ovary problems painful	sage *sage*	cypress camomile *cypress* juniper marjoram *melissa peppermint* rosemary	*jasmine marigold*
sterility (in women) vaginal irritation	bergamot	geranium melissa camomile	*jasmine* rose
Muscular aches and pains	*eucalyptus* sage thyme	black pepper camomile juniper *lavender* marjoram *rosemary*	
cramp lumbago rheumatism	basil eucalyptus lemon sage thyme	cypress marjoram camomile geranium camomile hyssop juniper lavender *marjoram rosemary*	camphor marigold
sprains	eucalyptus	hyssop lavender marjoram rosemary rosemary	
stiffness lack of tone	thyme lemongrass	black pepper lavender rosemary	
Nervous anxiety (panic)	basil bergamot thyme	camomile juniper lavender geranium majoram mellisa	cedarwood frankincense neroli rose

Problem	Top Notes	Middle Notes	Base Notes
apathy			jasmine
depression	basil bergamot clary sage *thyme*	rosemary *camomile* geranium lavender	*camphor* frankincense *jasmine* neroli patchouli rose sandalwood ylang-ylang
excitability (keyed up)	lemon sage thyme	*camomile* cypress hyssop juniper lavender marjoram	neroli ylang-ylang
insomnia	basil	camomile juniper lavender marjoram	camphor neroli rose sandalwood ylang-ylang
irritability		camomile cypress lavender marjoram	neroli rose
nervous debility (run down)	*basil* clary sage *sage*	lavender juniper marjoram	benzoin *jasmine* marigold
nervous tension (anxiety)	basil bergamot clary sage thyme	camomile geranium juniper *lavender* *marjoram* melissa	*jasmine* marigold *neroli* rose sandalwood ylang-ylang
neuralgia (facial)	eucalyptus	*camomile geranium* peppermint	
neuralgia (rheumatic)	eucalyptus	camomile hyssop lavender marjoram	
shock		melissa peppermint	camphor neroli
stress		juniper	cedarwood *neroli* rose
Obesity cellulite		fennel juniper lavender rosemary	

Problem	Top Notes	Middle Notes	Base Notes
congestion fluid retention	lemon sage	geranium rosemary cypress fennel geranium juniper lavender rosemary	patchouli
oedema	eucalyptus sage	geranium juniper	
Respiratory asthma	basil lemon sage thyme	cypress *hyssop lavender* marjoram melissa peppermint *pine rosemary*	benzoin
bronchitis	basil bergamot *eucalyptus* lemon sage	hyssop *lavender* melissa peppermint *pine* rosemary	benzoin sandalwood
catarrh	basil eucalyptus lemon thyme	black pepper *hyssop* lavender marjoram peppermint	cedarwood frankincense jasmine myrrh sandalwood
coughs	*eucalyptus thyme*	black pepper *cypress hyssop* lavender rosemary	benzoin cedarwood jasmine myrrh
emphysema	basil *eucalyptus thyme*	cypress *hyssop*	jasmine
flu	*eucalyptus lemon* sage *thyme*	camomile *cypress* hyssop *lavender* peppermint pine rosemary	benzoin camphor sandalwood
(preventative) hay fever		fennel hyssop	
hiccough	basil	fennel	

Problem	Top Notes	Middle Notes	Base Notes
Scalp			
alopecia (hair loss)	*sage* thyme	*lavender* rosemary	cedarwood
dandruff		rosemary	cedarwood
scurf	lemon	camomile geranium	cedarwood
seborrhoea		juniper	
Skin			
acne	lemongrass	camomile *juniper* lavender	*camphor* cedarwood
allergy prone and sensitive		camomile	jasmine neroli rose
animal bites	sage	lavender	myrrh
boils	lemon thyme	camomile lavender	marigold neroli rose
broken capillaries	lemon	camomile cypress	
		lavender peppermint	
bruises	sage	fennel hyssop marjoram	camphor marigold
		marjoram	
burns	eucalyptus sage	camomile geranium	camphor marigold
		lavender rosemary	
chapped and cracked		camomile geranium	*benzoin patchouli*
			rose sandalwood
congested	basil sage	geranium peppermint	
		rosemary	
dermatitis	sage	camomile hyssop	benzoin
		geranium juniper lavender	

Problem	Top Notes	Middle Notes	Base Notes
dry		camomile lavender geranium	jasmine neroli rose sandalwood ylang-ylang
eczema (general)	sage	camomile hyssop	
(dry)		geranium lavender	
(weeping)	bergamot	juniper	
herpes	bergamot eucalyptus lemon	geranium lavender	frankincense marigold myrrh rose sandalwood
inflamed	clary sage	camomile lavender	
insect bites and stings	basil lemon sage thyme	geranium peppermint *lavender* melissa	cedarwood
insect repellent	basil *eucalyptus*	geranium peppermint	cedarwood jasmine neroli sandalwood
irritable (less than 1% i.e. 5 drops in 50ml)		peppermint	
mature	clary sage	cypress lavender	benzoin frankincense myrrh neroli patchouli rose
mouth ulcers and thrush	lemon sage	geranium	*myrrh*
oily (open pores)	bergamot *lemon*	cypress geranium *juniper* lavender	camphor *cedarwood ylang-ylang*
psoriasis	bergamot	lavender	*frankincense jasmine* marigold myrrh neroli patchouli
rejuvenating and regenerating	lemon	*lavender* melissa	
sunburn		lavender	
super sensitive		camomile	jasmine neroli rose

Problem	Top Notes	Middle Notes	Base Notes
wounds	bergamot *eucalyptus* thyme	*camomile* geranium hyssop juniper *lavender* rosemary	benzoin camphor frankincense *myrrh* patchouli
Special arthritis bed wetting	lemon *sage* thyme	*camomile* juniper cypress	*benzoin*
cancer (prevention and treatment)	bergamot sage	cypress geranium *hyssop*	
gout	basil	camomile fennel *juniper* pine rosemary	*benzoin*
sweating (perspiration)	bergamot clary sage sage	cypress pine	

13.

Case Histories

It is always exciting and stimulating to read about successful case histories, but at the same time it must be remembered that for every ten spectacular cases there are ten with only mediocre results and possibly one or two on whom very little change is noticed. These are the people who probably need another form of natural treatment as back up such as acupuncture, reflexology, diet or naturopathy. Also, if *only* the symptoms are being treated, or if it is not clear what is *causing* the symptoms and therefore the wrong choice of oil is made, then the results cannot be expected to be miraculous. Don't give up, try a different mix of essential oils.

I have one case history myself (not yet complete) of just such a happening. The daughter of a friend of mine was having problems with recurring eczema in 1981 and wanted to try a natural remedy. I mixed her an eczema cream and she was delighted with the results. She has been clear enough to only need her second pot in 1982, twelve months later. A few weeks ago she rang me to ask if I could mix something for her boyfriend who had a 'sort of prickly heat' rash for a few weeks and the irritation was getting him down. So I mixed him an oil containing peppermint and sandalwood ... I didn't see Hazel for a while but when I did she said it hadn't done a lot for his rash. It did lessen the irritation, but it wasn't clearing up. After further conversation (not having ever seen him, by the way!) I came to the conclusion that it may be a type of contact dermatitis, and suggested that I see him before mixing any further oils. This was only three days ago so I haven't yet been able to try another remedy.

★   ★   ★

A client of mine, Mrs F of Hinckley, whom I met when giving a talk on aromatherapy at a ladies night in 1982, did not have success on my first attempt to clear up the blotchy, dry skin on her face. I first of all gave her normal Essentia for a dry skin, and after four days her skin was no better, but even drier than before! (I must add here that she had been using a mineral oil based moisturizer, which tends to draw moisture from below your skin surface as well as the air, in order to keep the surface moist, so without that her skin was extra dry.) I then asked her to take her moisture cream into work and apply it every two hours, and she came to the salon where I gave her a face mask to stimulate the blood circulation. After a week she rang me up to say that it was back to 'normal' and no longer extra dry but it was still blotchy and as dry as when I first met her. Not many ladies would have persevered as Susan did, and I am very grateful to her for that, as I really wanted to get to the bottom of it. She came again to the salon, where my husband, who is a trichologist (and covered diseases of the skin in his training) asked if there was any history of eczema, asthma or hay fever in her family. 'Yes' was the answer – though she herself had no symptoms – whereupon Len suggested I mix a moisture cream containing oils for treating eczema. This I did, and a delighted Mrs F came in to see me two weeks later, with a lovely clear and soft skin – no blotches or dry patches. Needless to say she has been using this special moisture cream ever since.

I am really grateful for her perseverance; many would have just assumed themselves allergic to this new product and gone back to the other one, without contacting me and giving me a chance to try something else. The *only* difference between the first moisture cream she tried and the second was in the essential oils I used. Now, whenever I meet anyone with a problem like Mrs F's, I always ask about the eczema, asthma or hay fever link, and so far I have had great success. I call it my 'Special E' cream, and the range includes night cream, hand lotion, after bath lotion, massage oil and sun tan lotion. Mrs F uses the normal cleanser for dry skin because that doesn't stay on the skin for long, but is washed off.

*   *   *

Mrs U, also of Hinckley, had a hip replacement nearly four years ago. This didn't 'take' and after many complications and a lot of pain she has had the replacement removed. The skin on her leg is very dry since the operation, so she uses an Essentia After Bath Lotion with special oils in it, which keeps her skin from flaking. The arthritic oil I mixed for her has helped the pain in her hands and shoulders considerably, and a few weeks ago I mixed her an oil for bruises as the slightest knock comes up in a bruise. I am about to give her an oil now to help to reduce the scar tissue on her thigh. It is actually an oil to prevent stretch marks but I have had success with stretch marks *after* pregnancy with this particular mix of essential oils, in 1978, on someone who didn't take care *during* pregnancy to prevent stretch marks appearing in the first place.

★   ★   ★

Judy, one of my staff, used my anti-stretch mark oil all during her pregnancy two years ago in 1980, and because she was so delighted has recommended it to Kay, another girl on my staff who has just become pregnant. Marlene, who tested the stretch mark oil on her six year old stretch marks in 1979 also tested an oil I made for cellulite and fluid retention, with results that were sufficient for her husband to notice the difference on her thighs.

★   ★   ★

Mrs L from Hinckley is using this same oil for fluid retention in her ankles She was having to take two water tablets a day and the continual visits to the toilet were making her feel weak and miserable. After one week of massaging the Essentia oil into her lower legs and feet, her ankles had gone down about one inch (2½ cm) in circumference. She told her doctor, because she was so delighted (he is my doctor too!) and he laughed, saying 'Ah, yes, Shirley and her ideas — it won't do you any harm, anyway!' Mrs Lowe is now only taking *one* water tablet a day and her ankles have stayed less swollen. This is about eight weeks later.

★   ★   ★

A client of mine has a young 8 year old with eczema. Caroline puts the lotion on herself, and whenever the eczema appears it will clear up when she uses her special cream. Her mother has now asked me to mix something for her own lack of muscle tone. A few weeks ago she came to my salon for a course of electrical facial treatments to rejuvenate tired and dry skins. I recommended using the creams accompanying the treatment at home between each visit, which she did, and liked them very much. Unfortunately they proved too expensive to keep up, so I suggested she try my Essentia range, with essential oils to treat dry and lined skin. She swears her skin is even better than before and I must admit that the frankincense in Essentia night cream has done wonders for her neck.

* * *

Mrs F is a client who suffers from psoriasis. This is a difficult problem to treat as it returns from time to time. Mrs F started using Essentia Psoriasis Hand Lotion about two years ago and finds that with regular daily use she never has a severe breakout like she used to have.

* * *

Penny, my own daughter who is now 26, had a nervous rash four years ago which left her with severe irritation all over her body in cold weather. A mixture of sandalwood and peppermint in the right proportions was a great help to her at these times, keeping the irritation at bay. As soon as her nervous problem was resolved the 'symptoms' (i.e., the rash) disappeared altogether and she no longer needed the oils. When she was better, we then tackled her period problems. She did not begin to menstruate until she was 16, and then very spasmodically, sometimes going for as long as seven months without a period. She also had a weight problem from about the same age and used to fast for three or four days at a time, drinking only liquids. She did this because if she exceeded 500 calories a day she put on weight! Then she would get fed up and nibble one or two biscuits with her coffee on a 'fasting' day, and of course her weight was never stable. Last summer in 1981, when she was on vacation from college, we decided to tackle the periods with essential oils, and she had an oil to massage on her tummy, and a neat essential oil mix for her bath, every other day. Within a week she had a period, and we continued with the treatment for the rest of the twelve weeks. Six weeks later she had another period and they are now coming every four or five weeks without using the oils. *BUT*, one of the biggest benefits was that after the periods began to come regularly she shed her surplus weight, now eats normally (but eats no butter, though a lot of bran and fibre) and is a size 12, to her own and our delight!

Cramp is another problem which is very easily helped with essential oils. I haven't yet had a failure with it. My first success was Mrs P of Sharnford, who suffered badly with cramp during the night. I mixed her an oil to massage into her left foot and calf each night for the first week and once a week thereafter, and a bath oil to put into her bath once a week. She has never had cramp since and that was two and a half years ago. She is just off to Australia to live with her daughter and is taking a year's supply with her!

*   *   *

Brenda is a client of mine who also acts as a model for me when I am teaching aromatherapy to other people on my courses. She had severe cramp pains in the toes of her left foot. I gave her 'a magic little bottle of oils' (in Brenda's own words) 'and even after two nights the pain had almost disappeared. At the first sign of recurrence of pain I only have to use it for one night and it disappears.'

*   *   *

My friend Iris from Earl Shilton also suffered from cramp, but no longer does. Her husband used the same oil for his sprained knee and fortunately the marjoram in Iris's oil was the essential oil for sprains too — though neither knew that at the time he used it! I have since mixed an oil for her mother-in-law for rheumatism, and an insect repellant for her daughter, who went to Africa this year on holiday! Last year, Iris asked me if I could do anything for her sinuses — she was considering an operation, but would prefer to try aromatherapy first, just in case it might help. In her own words, 'I have suffered from sinusitis for several years, with frequent severe attacks, especially during the winter. My face was often swollen and painful along the cheek bone, and I suffered with headaches. In the winter of '81/82 the condition was very persistent so in January '82 I asked Shirley if she could help. She gave me an oil for putting in the bath and an oil for massaging into the face, with detailed instructions about the pressure to do along the area of the sinus blockage.'

'Initially I used the bath oil two or three times a week, now only once a week. The massage oil was used initially every night. After four weeks I had considerable relief from the condition. Shirley then suggested that instead of using Essentia night cream with the oils in for skin rejuvenation, I should use one with oils in for sinus problems. I use this every night, as I did the other night cream, but when I get a cold I use the massage oil with my pressures.'

'Result – the condition is greatly improved, even with a cold; it seems able to prevent mucous congesting, and I haven't had a severe attack ever since.'

★   ★   ★

Mr C, a patient of my husband, who is a trichologist, complained of scalp eruptions and intense irritation. Having tried one of his trichology lotions without total success, my husband asked me if I could suggest one of my oils. I made up a base cream with the eczema oils in it form him to try (pure guess work!) and there was an instant improvement. One 100g pot was sufficient to return his scalp to normal, though he had to use Len's special shampoo to keep it clear.

★   ★   ★

Mrs J came to see Len with similar eruptions on her face and many tiny lumps under the skin surface. Any skin product irritated the condition, so Len asked me if I could mix her a face moisturizer for use after washing. Again it was the eczema oils which brought success.

★   ★   ★

Hair loss is a difficult condition to treat, but I have found that regular *correct* massage definitely prevents further thinning, and in quite a number of cases actually revives hair follicles which have lost the ability to produce hair. When this massage is preceded by the application of carrier oil containing rosemary and cedarwood the texture of the hair is improved and thickening is noticeable after six to eight months of *regular* weekly use. Cases are too numerous to mention, but at least eight women and five men have benefited from this treatment and names will be supplied on request.

★   ★   ★

The following case histories, which have been sent to me by practising aromatherapists and reflexologists whom I have trained, have not been re-written. I have included their names in Useful Addresses at the back of the book so that should you live in their area and require professional treatment and help you can contact them.

*   *   *

From Mrs Teresa Silva, now practising in Spain, whom I trained in July, 1982:

I would inform you that Miss P was involved in a nasty car accident about five years ago. Her back and neck got knocked about over this accident. For two years she has been unable to resume her work, and lead a normal life. However for the past three years she has been coping, although unable to sleep through one night without interrupting, due to pain in her neck.

Another complaint was the lack of punctuality over her period cycle, and the swelling over her tummy. She also suffers considerably of constipation.

On the 25th August, I gave her my first treatment using the following oils: Melissa, Marjoram, Lavender, Juniper.

On the 26th August, she telephoned me at 10 a.m. excitedly to inform me that for the first time in a very long period she had slept right through the night. Moreover, her period was right on time, and also there was no constipation.

On the 3rd September (second treatment) she is still sleeping normal, the pain on her neck has subsided, and is now much more bearable, although there is still some tenderness in her tummy.

I shall endeavour to enquire further from her prior to seeing you on the 20th.

*   *   *

From Keith and Terry Clarke, Ryodoraku Acupuncture Clinic and Jasmine Beauty Clinic in Lincoln:

Here in Lincoln City Centre, where we run Jasmine Beauty Clinic alongside Ryodoraku Acupuncture Clinic, an experiment combining a course of aromatherapy in conjunction with acupuncture treatments, in cases of either severe arthritis or stress, has proved to be very successful. So much so, that our clients have returned after completion of treatments, requesting aromatherapy for the pure enjoyment of it. The following case-histories were particularly rewarding:

Case 'A' paid us a visit in May/June 1982 requesting acupuncture treatment for severe arthritis in the bottom of her spine, also in her hips. Her trouble had begun in December/January, since when she had been unable to walk any distance without pain, had difficulty in getting in and out of a chair, and was unable to sleep. Acupuncture was prescribed twice weekly for the first month, during which time the condition improved enough for an aromatherapy course to be introduced. The oils to be used were of Lavender, Benzoin, Rosemary. Both the acupuncture and the aromatherapy treatments were given at the rate of once per week for approximately three weeks. After which, both treatments were gradually reduced to once per month – alternating fortnightly. The lady in question is now, in the month of November 1982, 90 per cent free from her pain.

Case 'B' came to us in late August 1982 with severe pain resulting from an old disc problem. She had requested acupuncture treatment which of course was agreed upon. But we also suggested that it should be combined with a course of aromatherapy and this was also arranged – the oils used were of Rosemary, Benzoin, Lavender. Both treatments were given at intervals of approximately ten days, and our client gradually improved. In mid-October 1982, she had returned to work and now only calls upon us occasionally.

Case 'C' who had suffered severe neurosis for some considerable period of time, contacted us for acupuncture treatment in July of 1982 to help her condition. After discussing her problem at great length, it was agreed that the treatment would be carried out in the surroundings of her own home. It was necessary to treat her twice weekly for approximately three weeks before introducing a course of aromatherapy, again in conjunction with the acupuncture. The oils used were of Camomile, Juniper, Marjoram, Lavender. The initial treatments were at intervals of approximately five or six days. After her second aromatherapy, our client became much more able to relax, and both the aromatherapy and acupuncture treatments were gradually reduced to fortnightly visits. Although still undergoing treatments – this is November 1982 – our client is now able to travel to our clinic for a monthly visit. This is, of course, nearing the completion of all her treatments.

From Doreen Bader of Gt. Doddington, Northants, who also gives treatments in a local hospital:

Mr T, who was experiencing general tension, scalp tight, circulation poor in feet, indigestion problems. I used Ylang Ylang and Rosemary for his face; Lavender, Bergamot and Juniper for the body. I massaged Mr T once a week for five consecutive weeks and after that period (in fact well before) he was sleeping far better and relaxing and in fact he was able to leave off taking sleeping tablets and Valium.

Mrs B had very bad rheumatism in the feet and hands. I did massage on these areas over a four week period and she was able to actually move her toes (which before she was unable to do) and her hands were more flexible and less painful. I used for the massage Sage, Rosemary and Lavender.

Ms T had very badly swollen legs and ankles, and had had treatment at the local hospital — physiotherapy — which had not helped at all. I have been massaging this lady's legs and ankles twice a week over a four week period and even after the first two sessions there was a noticeable reduction in the swellings. She is now delighted to be able to see her ankle bones and her legs are now the normal size too (there were unsightly bumps before which have now gone down). I used for this lady Sage, Rosemary and Lavender.

Publisher' Note
In previous impressions of this book a brief account is included of aromatherapy treatment given to Mrs Jane George, a client of Doreen Bader, and we would like to record that the assessment of her condition and speculation as to the cause were the personal views of Doreen Bader and in no way represented the reason for Mrs George's visit to Doreen Bader.

Ms B had a very painful knee and I used both Aromatherapy massage and massage on the knee reflex on the feet to help. This alleviated the pain.

Ms W had pain around the sciatic nerve and I massaged her feet around this area (also part of the leg) and she has not had a recurrence!

Siobhann, currently working in the Bridge Beauty Salon in Coventry:

Mrs B had kidney problems, tension and cough. When doing reflexology on the foot, the kidney was quite painful; this was pointed out to the client, which confirmed her suspicions that she did in fact have a weak kidney. This client also suffered from bronchitis. When Mrs B returned home, after the massage treatment using Eucalyptus and Lavender, she slept for a good deal of the afternoon which is quite out of character. When she awoke she found that her breathing was not as tight as it had been in the past, and the niggling pain from her kidney had gone.

Mrs M: bronchitis and poor circulation
Treatment: Eucalyptus, Juniper.
When doing thumb pressure down the spine this client coughed continuously and I could feel all the nodules dispersing. A few hours after leaving the salon the client 'phoned to say that she had been able to unlodge all the mucous from her chest which then allowed her to breathe normally again.

Mrs H: cellulite, poor circulation
Treatment: Juniper.
This client is only having a leg massage as she is very embarrassed about the cellulite in her thighs. She is a very independent lady by nature and felt quite disgusted with herself for allowing them to reach this condition and not be able to treat them herself. She then sought the help of aromatherapy and I am working on the drainage principle. After about three weeks a visible difference was noticed which gave the client the confidence and will power to continue the treatment, therefore giving her the confidence in herself. Now, after ten weeks there is a great improvement in the condition of her thighs.

★　　　★　　　★

From Janice Benham (now Morgan) a mobile aromatherapist in Nottinghamshire:

Miss C, 18 years old. Backache that had lasted approximately two months had started through heavy lifting as this is part of her job. The doctor could not help her except to give painkillers and the suggestion to take things easy.

She came to me and I examined her back thoroughly and found that there were no vertebrae out of place. I then proceeded to do reflexology rather than back massage. The most tender spots were the lower back on both feet and the sciatic nerve affecting the hip. These areas were massaged on the feet for about fifteen minutes until they were hardly painful. I gave her a special oil to put'into the bath mixed mainly with Juniper and Rosemary. Another appointment was made for the following week. The next day Miss C was in a lot more pain in her back; the day after that the back was completely free from pain and stayed like that. When she came to me the following week she was completely pain free whereas before she had to miss work and was in tears because of the pain. I saw her recently six weeks after her last treatment and she was still pain free and had been able to go about her normal duties of work unhindered!

Mr C, a County Cricket Club captain could not bowl since the beginning of February, and it was now nearing the end of May. Everyone had said that he had neck trouble with not being able to twist his arm around for bowling; he also had terrible headaches. An osteopath, physiotherapist and acupuncturist had all been treating him since February for his neck.

On my first treatment of him I found that there were tender spots on his neck, head and also in his middle back (of which he was quite surprised). After this first treatment he found that his neck was much easier. I saw him for about three times a week over four weeks for about twenty minutes of reflexology each time. At first he and the physiotherapist were puzzled that I kept finding a problem spot in the middle back. The physiotherapist had a more careful look down the back and did find that there was a weakness in a disc in the middle back which was causing the neck and headache problems.

Slowly he started practising bowling as he felt fit. About three weeks after I had started treatment he bowled for the first time in a match and he did fantastically; the newspapers all commented on his performance.

If it had not been for reflexology the problem might never have been found and solved. Now the physiotherapist knows where to massage; rather than just concentrating on the neck he is mainly massaging the back and so far the problem has not returned.

One elderly woman came with osteoarthritis. Her right ankle was also badly damaged; it had been broken and was badly bruised, with no movement in it whatsoever. She also had a form of diabetes and was taking tablets for it. She came twice a week for fifteen minutes reflexology treatments for a few weeks and always had a bad reaction afterwards. Eventually though she was able to have longer treatments at longer intervals. Essential oils were also used made into bath oil and also body oil. Eventually one was found that helped immediately and that was a mixture of Camphor, Rosemary and Eucalyptus. The diet was also changed to Acid-Alkaline balanced.

There is now no bruise on her right ankle and it has a lot more movement. Her arthritis has been greatly improved and she feels very well inside. (Once, after one reflexology treatment, she said that she felt like running, she felt so well!). Her diabetes has improved and is now on reduced dosage of the tablets.

One of my clients, an elderly man, had advanced cancer of the bones and prostate gland. He also had arthritis and high blood pressure. He was taking drugs for the cancer and high blood pressure, plus 500 mg of aspirin every day.

At first I did not know if I could do anything to help him and he understood this but was quite willing to have a try. I found in reflexology that the whole body was out of balance, so I was very careful treating for about ten minutes each time on average twice a week. He dropped the aspirin straight away at commencement of the treatment. During three months of treatment he had stopped taking drugs for high blood pressure because the doctor had announced that it was now normal (it has stayed that way). He has never taken any aspirin since the start of the treatment.

Most of his tablets used to restrict his cancer have been stopped by the doctor. Generally his pain, although still there, is much improved; he used to walk with a walking stick which he does not need now. He has put on a lot of weight and looks quite sprightly and fit now. He is constantly improving as much as his age will allow.

There were other factors involved as well as reflexology. An aromatherapy oil was made up to help his aches and pains and also bath oil. His diet was also changed to acid-alkaline balanced. A very good multivitamin tablet, plus vitamin C (2 gm daily) is being taken.

Another client came to me very nervous, tense but with no real medical problem. I decided that the best course of treatment would be aromatherapy treatments, so full aromatherapy was given using calmative oils.

She felt much more relaxed for a long while afterwards, and now whenever she feels as though she is slipping back immediately books for an aromatherapy massage.

One client regularly comes for aromatherapy treatments about every six weeks. She finds that the aromatherapy keeps all her aches and pains at bay for a few weeks, plus making her feel well inside. In between treatments she uses the aromatherapy bath oil, which I make up similar to that which she has in her treatment.

There is one woman who I see once every so often when she feels depressed from personal problems more than anything else. She just has reflexology treatments whenever she needs them, and I generally see her about once every three months.

★   ★   ★

From June Ronald who practises aromatherapy in Milngavie, near Glasgow: (case histories written by her husband).

Mrs A had suffered from sinusitis for years and had tried various cures from her G.P. – medicines, sprays and more recently nasal syringes. She had experienced considerable relief after one aromatherapy treatment. Client was also given advice on how to use essential oils at home, and has since been feeling better than she has for years.

Miss B had been suffering from insomnia for some years, and has been taking tranquillizers constantly. After one aromatherapy she slept regularly and soundly every night of the following week without drugs.

Miss C was overweight though not obese. Excess weight was mainly in the form of cellulite. After a course of aromatherapy treatments the cellulite and hence her overall weight was considerably reduced.

Mrs D, aged 36, had failed to menstruate for six months though the pain continued, she felt depressed, and her weight increased. Advised by G.P. that this was due to menopause, her condition was diagnosed by aromatherapist as being due to a blockage, and after one aromatherapy treatment menstruation began the following day and associated problems quickly disappeared.

'Miss E, aged 22, came for treatment three weeks before her wedding, unable to cope with pre-nuptial pressures. After two aromatherapy treatments client felt and looked much better and was reported to be a 'radiant bride' on the big day.'

'Miss F suffered from pain in her right side. Her G.P. was only able to prescribe pain killers. Aromatherapist diagnosed a kidney condition. The client was advised to drink plenty of water and after a few aromatherapy treatments the pain had abated considerably.'

★   ★   ★

From Jackie Robertson and Brenda Etherington at Nordic Health and Sauna Centre, Whitley Bay, Tyne and Wear:

Name: Mrs L.

Diagnosis: Client suffers from extreme tension due to pressure of work, aches and muscular pains in lumbar region of back due to bending and lifting at work throughout the day. There is congestion in the back especially the lung area, due to heavy smoking. Client also suffers from cramp and an extremely dry skin, especially hands as they are always wet due to arranging flowers at work.

Treatment: The client came in at two week intervals and now comes in regularly every month.

Oils used: Juniper, lavender, sandalwood (avocado oil was added for quick penetration and for nourishment to skin).

Result: After the first treatment the client remarked that she felt as though a great weight had been lifted off her shoulders and head, and she felt very rested and relaxed. On her second visit she had been very busy at work putting in long hours and her whole body was aching. As I worked through the massage with more concentration on the knees and hands, she remarked that as I finished that particular part it ceased to ache. Client was given creams and oils for home use, mainly for dry skin and cramp, and has found a great improvement in general well-being and is more relaxed at work.

Name: Mrs M.

Diagnosis: Client was found to have bad circulation and congestion in lumbar region of back, mainly the right side where it was found that client suffers from arthritis in right hip. Due to the pain and discomfort of the arthritis the client was unable to get a restful night's sleep. The client is very fond of knitting and has knitted for many years for family and friends, and suffers from rheumatism in the joints of her hands, so being unable to knit for long. Client was also suffering from migraine headaches, found to be caused by the glasses she wore.

Treatment: Client came in each week for three weeks, and now comes in monthly.

Oils used: Eucalyptus, rosemary, sage.

Result: Client found great improvement in her general well-being and health. There was great ease in the right hip and client found much more restful nights and a great deal more movement of the whole right hip and leg. Knitting was much easier as the rheumatic pains in her hands had been alleviated. Client found that cold and damp weather affected her bad hip so a cream was made up for home use, and client has ceased to be bothered with hip.

Name: Mr M.

Diagnosis: Client had given his left knee a knock, causing it to swell and causing discomfort and loss of movement. Client was also suffering from pains all over back but more so in lumbar region, first thought to be due to work. But after a consultation with his doctor he was found to have 'Sherman's disease' for which there is no known cure. Client was very tense due to work and also the discomfort of his back. Client has suffered from sinus since childhood. Due to overnight travelling through work he was suffering from insomnia and eyestrain.

Oils used: Sage, juniper, lavender, jasmine.

Result: At the beginning of treatment the client was very tense and unable to relax, but after some gentle reassurance the client became so relaxed he could be moved like a puppet. There was found to be much ease in the back and the swelling in the knee went down. The client also found breathing much easier. The client was given oils and creams for home use. A bath oil and body lotion to use nightly for his back; he has found great ease, for the pain has been alleviated and he is able to work much better. Also a cream for his sinus problem; he has found breathing easier.

★   ★   ★

Useful Addresses

Essential Oil Suppliers

Shirley Price
Sketchley Manor
Burbage
Leics. LE10 2LQ
(Also supplies the Essentia
Skin Care range)

The Birch Twig
80 Castle Street
Hinckley
Leics. LE10 1DD
(Also supplies ready mixed
treatment oils)

Purple Flame
61 Clinton Lane
Kenilworth
Warks.

H.O.F.
The Grange
Beaston Green
Sandy
Beds.

Field and Co (Aromatics) Ltd
Stonefield Close
South Ruislip
Middlesex

Index